Nutritional Wisdom, Plain and Simple

How to Lose Weight and Look and Feel Your Very Best

David Klein

Contents

Praise For *Nutritional Wisdom, Plain and Simple: How to Lose Weight and Look and Feel Your Very Best*

"Welcome to a journey of nutritional clarity and vitality! In this book, David Klein offers straightforward guidance on navigating the often confusing world of food choices. From debunking myths about common foods to unlocking the secrets of optimal meal timing and mindful eating, this book equips you with practical tools for enhancing your health and well-being. Discover the wisdom of the world's Blue Zones, learn effective strategies for weight loss, and embark on a path toward a healthier, happier you. I'm genuinely excited for this book and encourage all readers to explore its contents. May you find immense value and inspiration within these pages as you journey toward optimal health and vitality. Your natural partner in health, Dr. Linda Khoshaba, NMD, FABNE"

Dr. Khoshaba is the founder and director of Natural Endocrinology Specialists™ (NES), based in Scottsdale, Arizona, USA. She is a Board-Certified physician in Naturopathic Endocrinology.

"David Klein's 'Nutritional Wisdom Plain and Simple' is an essential guide that demystifies nutrition with clarity and practicality. Covering everything from proteins, fats, and carbohydrates to mindful eating and meal timing, Klein separates myths from facts, making complex concepts accessible to all. This book delves into various food types, the importance of gut health, and the impact of sleep on diet, providing a holistic approach to eating well. Perfect for anyone looking to enhance their health, it's a comprehensive resource you'll turn to again and again."

Jennifer Tardy, Certified Holistic Nutritionist, Integrative Health Coach, Certified Weight Loss Specialist, Fitness and Nutrition Program Designer, and Owner of Eating for Healing Nutrition & Wellness.

Acknowledgements

My heart goes out to all of those who have always wanted to be trim and healthy but have never known how to do so. As Dr. Joel Fuhrman so reasonably points out, our early education should be reading, writing, arithmetic, and nutrition. Sadly, we were never taught proper nutrition, and commercial forces have created an environment that works against our health. May you find redemption in the information in this book, and may you always enjoy better food and better health.

To Dr. Linda Khoshaba. Thank you for your kind words about this book and your helpful guidance and compassion. May your practice continue to thrive.

To nutritionist Jennifer Tardy. Thank you, Jennifer, for your help and kind guidance that helped me to make final decisions and complete this book. Your knowledge of the field of nutrition is remarkable.

To Betty Swain. You are one of the most lovely people we have ever known—you possess a beautiful and generous spirit. We think of you often, and we look forward to the good times ahead.

And, to my favorite person in the world . . . my dear wife Rae. You amaze me. Your qualities absolutely shine with stunning brilliance. What a beautiful bright spot you have been, and I cherish you dearly. As I mention in every book . . . you are hilarious—the funniest person I know, and you really crack me up. And if you don't mind me telling the world . . . I really, really like you!

Introduction

"The world of diet and nutrition can be overwhelming and filled with misinformation and inaccurate health claims." So wrote Shanley Chienthe, senior health editor at U.S. News. And she is correct. People are confused, and they don't know what to eat, how to eat, or when to eat.

Likely you've been confused too. Most of us have. We've bounced from diet to diet and from one nutritional strategy to the next. For most of us, we are still searching for answers, because what we've been doing has not worked. In recent decades, we've collectively become more overweight and more plagued with disease. Obesity and conditions like diabetes are at an all-time high and are still on the rise. But it doesn't need to be that way. When we cut through the confusion and apply wisdom to the field of nutrition, it's all really simple and our health outcomes are good. We just need to learn what to do.

Dr. Joel Fuhrman, who is a leader in the field of health and nutrition and the founder of the Nutritarian diet, makes this point clear in his book *The End of Dieting*. Discussing the diet industry, he wrote: "Our collective dietary ignorance is the only thing keeping that industry alive. If people understood the basic principles of nutritional excellence, they would understand that they need to eat healthfully, and by doing so they would achieve their ideal weight and never feel compelled to diet again. They wouldn't jump from one popular diet book to another looking for a quick fix. They wouldn't have to."

And that is why I wrote this book. My promise to you is to clear up the nutritional confusion in the diet industry and teach you the principles of sound nutritional excellence. I've spent years diligently studying the works of the best minds in the field of nutrition from all around the world. In many ways, this book is a compilation of their combined expertise and wisdom.

In part one of this book, you'll learn the principles of truly wise nutrition. You'll learn *what to eat*, including all you need to know about each of the three macronutrients: protein, carbohydrates, and fats, including how much of each you should eat.

I'll clear up the confusion regarding such often controversial foods as dairy, meat, eggs, olive oil, beans, grains, and others. Are they healthy foods, or are they not? Should you include them in your diet? And if so, how much of them should you eat?

You'll learn how to improve your all-important microbiome, and you'll learn how to supplement wisely.

You'll also learn *when to eat,* which some consider almost as important as what to eat. Specifically, you'll learn about meal timing, eating in harmony with your circadian rhythms, and time-restricted eating.

And finally, you'll learn *how to eat* more healthfully, including the amazing benefits gained from thorough chewing, mindful eating, and eating the right amount of food. You'll learn the way to be satiated, or satisfied, with lesser amounts of food.

In part two you'll learn about the world's five Blue Zones. In these regions, residents are extraordinarily healthy and live long and vibrant lives, frequently reaching the status of centenarian, or 100 years old. Residents in all five Blue Zones, even though spanning five countries and four continents, share common dietary patterns.

There is a wonderful section on weight loss, which teaches the best ways to lose weight safely and without distress. You'll learn how to stabilize your blood glucose, and I discuss a very interesting concept called "The Pleasure Trap." You'll learn how to avoid or escape that dangerous and destructive dietary trap. And you'll learn why all calories are not equal.

Part three is very brief, but it gets its own section because of its importance. In condensed detail, it outlines the healthiest diet in the world. Part three is essentially a summary, or cheat sheet, of all of the top wonderful concepts that you learned earlier in the book. Follow those 23 points and you will be sure to enjoy a boost in vitality and more robust health.

This book is about nutritional wisdom, plain and simple. There are no fad diets involved and no wacky recommendations—just solid and sound nutritional advice that is proven to work among the healthiest and most long-lived people in the world. I'm thrilled to be able to share this with you, and it's my hope that you benefit greatly and enjoy a huge boost to your health—and weight loss if you desire it—from the proven principles you'll be learning about. That's the benefit of understanding and applying sound nutritional wisdom. May you enjoy reading this book as much as I did writing it. The very best of health to you!

David Klein
June, 2024

How To View Changes You May Need to Make

This book is designed to give you an excellent education about healthy eating and to clear up any nutritional confusion that you may have. But more importantly, it's also designed to empower you to make any dietary changes that will help you to improve your health and your life. But how should you view those changes? How far should you go with them? The information here may help you to get a better grasp of that before you dive into the good stuff ahead.

Let's start with a little story I'd like to share with you, which is the supposed transcript between United States and Canadian sea captains off the coast of Newfoundland in October, 1995, in a mini-battle of wits:

Americans: "Please divert your course 15 degrees to the North to avoid a collision."

Canadians: "Recommend you divert your course 15 degrees to the South to avoid a collision."

Americans: "This is the captain of a US Navy ship. I say again, divert your course."

Canadians: "No, I say again, you divert your course."

Americans: "We are getting closer. Now you need to divert your course 30 degrees to the North."

Canadians: "Now you need to divert your course 30 degrees to the South."

Americans: "This is now urgent . . . Now you need to divert your course 45 degrees to the North."

Canadians: "You immediately need to divert your course 45 degrees to the South."

Americans: "THIS IS THE AIRCRAFT CARRIER USS ABRAHAM LINCOLN, THE SECOND LARGEST SHIP IN THE UNITED STATES' ATLANTIC FLEET. WE ARE ACCOMPANIED BY THREE DESTROYERS, THREE CRUISERS AND NUMEROUS SUPPORT VESSELS. I DEMAND THAT YOU

CHANGE YOUR COURSE 45 DEGREES NORTH. THAT'S FOUR-FIVE DEGREES NORTH, OR COUNTER MEASURES WILL BE UNDERTAKEN TO ENSURE THE SAFETY OF THIS SHIP."

Canadians: "This is a lighthouse. Your call."

That's a great story, but a little research shows that it's likely not real; it was made up for entertainment purposes. Regardless, it teaches a great lesson, even in the matter of nutrition. The point: The lighthouse wins. It's not budging at all. It can't. And if success is to be had, and a collision avoided, that proud ship better take action, and sooner rather than later.

Likewise, our bodily needs are not going to change course for us. They can't. They are as firmly grounded and set as the lighthouse. If we want to live a longer life, enjoy vibrant health, and avoid obesity and serious health problems, we too will need to change course with what we eat, as well as perhaps when we eat and how we eat. Some of us will need to make a little 15-degree swerve, others might need a 30 or 45-degree adjustment, while others, those who are already in serious trouble or recognize that they are rapidly heading there, might need to do what almost amounts to a 180-degree turnaround, or close to it. I encourage you to be honest with yourself and make any changes that you believe are necessary.

And while I encourage you to be very diligent, I suggest you don't become fanatical. Make steady improvements to your diet, try things out, and as you see your health and life improve, you are likely going to want to continue on that same course. In the process, you will be continually gaining more skill in healthy eating.

Please note these wise words from Marty Kendall, who is an Australian engineer who has devoted his life's work to the study of and teaching about nutritional health, weight control, and longevity. In my opinion, he's done so beautifully and with great wisdom; he uses his engineering background to brilliantly conceptualize and explain nutritional principles. He writes: "Your diet doesn't need a name or a belief system, just nutrients!"

In this book, we'll be focusing on eating the proper nutrients you will need that will help your body to thrive.

Part 1: A Nutritional Primer, With Recommendations

What to Eat

Chapter 1

Why Fad Diets Do Not Work

• Fad diets have been the rage for as long as anyone can remember. It seems like a new fad diet is introduced every couple of months, and many jump on the bandwagon. Then, often as quickly as it came, the fad diet is gone. Why are fad diets so popular? Why do they fail?

Fad nutrition, including fad diets, are very popular. Some people jump from one fad diet to the next. That's sad, because, simply, fad nutrition and fad diets do not work.

If they don't work, why are they so popular?

There are several reasons. One of them, ironically, is that all of the other fad diets people have tried have failed. So, for them, they move on to the next one with hope renewed.

Fad diets are also usually overhyped. Those promoting such diets know how to push all of the right buttons to get people interested.

And here is the biggest reason that fad diets are so popular: they seem to work . . . at first.

There was one fad diet that was popular in my locality about five years ago. Many people I knew went on the diet and lost weight. Lots of it. And quickly. However, within just a year or two they all abandoned the diet and gained back at least as much weight as they lost . . . and they damaged their health in the process. (More on Yoyo dieting later in the book.)

Why would anyone have such success on a diet and then suddenly abandon it? The answer is that the diet is not sustainable. It promises and delivers short-term results, which tends to whip people into a frenzy. But then nutritional deficiencies from the structure of the diet begin to make the person feel unwell, and then sick, and then very sick, and they have no choice but to stop.

An extreme example of this is a long water fast. If you were to stop eating all food and just drink water for a time, you would lose weight and lose it quickly. That could be very encouraging each time you stepped on the scale. However, after a few days or so your body and brain would be screaming for food. The weight is still coming off, but the joy of the loss of weight is replaced by the stark reality and pain and emptiness of not eating at all. Simply, that is not sustainable.

Many other diets have a similar effect. Nutritionist Lindsay Christensen mentioned to me that many of her clients had been vegans. (For the record, I don't consider veganism to be a fad diet.) And they felt great for a while, with all of the plant nutrients that they were eating. However, certain nutrients are very difficult to obtain on a vegan diet, such as protein, vitamin B12, retinol, and omega-3 fatty acids. It can be done, including with supplementation, but it's not easy. And when those clients began to feel the effects of the nutritional deficiencies, they stopped veganism (but still ate lots of plant foods) and felt better.

Those who go on extreme low carb diets get a real "bonus" at the start of their diets that encourages them immensely. The bonus is that they lose weight rapidly in the first week or so. They may lose six pounds the first week. And then they begin the calculations . . . by losing six pounds a week they will be losing about 25 pounds a month. They need to lose 50 pounds, so, in their minds, two months should do it.

It doesn't. Not even close.

Here's what is happening. When someone starts a very low carb diet, they lose a little bit of fat, but they lose a lot of water weight. We all carry a certain amount of water in our bodies, and when carbohydrate intake is low, we'll shed water immediately. (Notice the word "hydrate" in carbohydrates.) But once that's happened, usually within a week, there's no more excess water weight to lose. From that point on, the weight loss might be one pound, not six pounds a week.

The extreme low carb dieter may be content losing one pound a week, which is actually a very good rate to lose weight, but the lack of carbohydrates and other nutrients that fresh fruits and other carb foods provide will begin to cause nutritional deficiencies. Again, a feeling of being unwell and sick takes over, and the person has no choice but to abandon the diet.

Some who have done so have gone ballistic with carbohydrates in the other direction. They've felt starved for carbs for so long, that now they can't seem to get enough of them—including refined carbohydrates. And when that happens, all of the water weight comes back in days, and then all of the lost fat soon returns too, often with extra "bonus" pounds.

The shortcomings of fad dieting were summed up nicely by the University of California at San Diego, Center for Healthy Eating and Activity Research. They wrote: "Any diet based on restricting specific food groups, combining foods in a specific order or timing, or following rigid menus each day are typically unsustainable and harmful to your health. Such diets show quick results, but not because you are losing fat. Fad diets target fiber, lean muscle, and water weight loss. This type of weight loss causes deficiencies to nutrition, dehydration, and fatigue."

You'll be happy to know that this book is fad free. Solid principles of sound nutrition are highlighted on every page. When you get the nutrition right, everything else seems to fall in place.

Macronutrients and Micronutrients

Macronutrients and micronutrients. What are they? Macronutrients refer to the three major sources of calories in our diets: proteins, carbohydrates, and fats. (Alcohol is also a source of calories, but it should never be a major source of calories, for obvious reasons.) Micronutrients refer to vitamins and minerals, which are vital for our overall health, well-being, and for disease prevention. Micronutrients cannot be produced in our bodies, so we must get them from our food. The only vitamin that can be produced in the body is vitamin D, through sun exposure on the skin. But vitamin D is not really a vitamin; it's a hormone.

It should be noted that in the plant kingdom, the vast majority of foods have a healthful mix of all three macronutrients. These beautiful combinations are one of the reasons that our foods taste so delicious. It's rare for a food to have just one macronutrient at the exclusion of the other two.

One macronutrient is not better than the others. They are all vital to our health, and they each have different functions. Each gram of protein and each gram of carbohydrates yields four calories, while each gram of fat yields nine calories.

We are not going to cover micronutrients in detail here, because they are too numerous to reasonably cover in a book of this nature. And please note that there is also a category called phytonutrients, or phytochemicals. These include carotenoids, polyphenols, flavonoids, lignans, and more. In fact, between 50,000 and 130,000 phytonutrients have been discovered, and we are definitely not going to list and discuss all those here. But the vastness of that number shows the precious value of eating natural foods. There's much in those foods that is meant to build and protect our health. Many benefits of phytonutrients are still being discovered.

And before we learn about each of the three macronutrients, please note that it is important to make sure that we are consuming reasonable proportions of those nutrients in our diets. But that doesn't mean that we need to compulsively count each gram of each macronutrient. Please note these wise words of Dr. Joel Fuhrman, a brilliant nutritional doctor and prolific author: "Whatever ratio of fat, protein, and carbohydrate you eat doesn't matter (within reason, of course). It is predominantly the nutritional quality and healthfulness of those carbs, fats, and proteins that determine your health." Always aim for nutritional quality, balance and reasonableness in your dietary patterns,

Chapter 2

Protein

● Protein has at times been referred to as the "king of the macronutrients." How much protein do we need in our diets for optimal health—low protein, high protein, or somewhere in between? Which is healthier, animal or plant protein? Do our protein requirements change as we age? What is protein leveraging, and why is it important?

What Does Protein Do, and Why Do We Need It in Our Diets?

The main function of protein in our diets is to build and maintain muscle mass and strength, as well as to repair muscles from the wear and tear of exercise and daily living. Carbs and fats are simply not designed to do this, so the entire burden falls on protein. Without adequate protein intake, our muscles would soon atrophy, and we'd be in big trouble . . . Remember, the heart is a muscle—and a weak heart does not equal vibrant health or a long life.

Proteins are formed by smaller compounds called amino acids. I like this succinct explanation by the government website medlineplus.gov: "Amino Acids are molecules that combine to form proteins. Amino acids and proteins are the building blocks of life."

There are twenty amino acids that combine to form the proteins that are necessary for life. Eleven of these are considered "nonessential" amino acids, and nine are considered "essential." What's the difference? Nonessential amino acids are those that can be made in our bodies, so it's not essential that we consume them in our diets. The nine essential amino acids are not produced in our bodies, so it's essential to our health that we get them from our food.

How Much Protein Do We Need in Our Diets?

How much protein should you be eating? To a large degree, that depends upon your own personal situation and needs, including your size, age, and your lifestyle, including your need for muscular strength. Smaller people need less protein, older people tend to need more protein, and those who are involved in sports or professions that require power also need more protein.

Some years ago, while living in Dallas, Texas, I was having a telephone conversation with my father, who lived out of state. I had recently been packing on the pounds, including muscle, which I mentioned to him. He asked what my current weight was, and I said 225. He then cleverly asked if I was playing linebacker for the Dallas Cowboys. Good question. With my sedentary work, and at my height of 6'0", I did not need to be carrying 225 pounds. (And I'm not anymore. By living according to the nutritional principles in this book, I'm back to my high school, college, and young adult weight of less than 160 pounds.)

I'll be discussing the Blue Zones regions later in this book, which are areas where residents live especially long lives, frequently into their 90s and 100s, at a much higher rate than in other localities. There are five identified Blue Zones in five different countries. They are Okinawa, Japan; Sardinia, Italy; Nicoya Peninsula, Costa Rica; Ikaria, Greece; and Loma Linda, California, United States. In the five Blue Zones, there is a common thread involving protein intake. Namely, residents tend to consume relatively low to moderate amounts of protein during their lifetimes. While they are not an especially muscular people, Blue Zones inhabitants have sufficient strength to work and socialize to the full every day and into the evening. Many work at such professions as shepherding, and they regularly walk several miles a day, even up and down hills and mountains, as they accomplish their tasks. Then they return home to eat, socialize, and dance with family and friends.

Their work, in a way, reminds me of the work of a United States delivery driver for a company such as Fed Ex or UPS. They both stay active and move around all day. That said, I would still guess that they would not have the same protein requirements. Why? Shepherding or caring for mountainside goats or tending a Mediterranean vineyard or olive grove is done at a rather relaxed pace—it's hard work but the pace is gentle on both the body and the mind. But the delivery drivers have to lift, frequently, very heavy packages, and it seems like their routes are pressure-packed—they are always charging on to the next destination. (Drivers sometimes run up to our door and run back to their trucks.) That additional stress, and wear and tear, would likely create the need for a higher amount of daily dietary protein.

Valter Longo, who is often considered the world's leading longevity research scientist, asks this relevant question: <u>"What is the lowest level of protein that you can take to get the muscles you need?"</u> And that is really the spot-on answer to how much protein you should consume. In other words, it's best to eat the amount of protein that you need and not much more.

As you can see, it's not possible to recommend an exact amount of protein, because each person has different needs, and your needs will also change over the course of your life. In a moment, I'll provide a general range. But in the meantime, keep in mind these words of wisdom by David Raubenheimer and Stephen J. Simpson, the authors of the book *Eat Like the Animals*: "Try adjusting up and down until you feel in control of your appetites—hungry by mealtimes and satisfied after and between meals." Actually, I encourage you to do this with other areas of your diet as well. Keep on experimenting until you find what works best for you, adjusting up and down as need be, honing in on what is ideal.

As to the comment "hungry by mealtimes and satisfied between meals," this is in harmony with the fact that it's a good idea to eat sufficient protein at breakfast. A minimum of 20 or 25 to 30 grams is usually a good target. If you eat too little protein at breakfast and too many carbs, especially high-glycemic carbs, your blood glucose will rise quickly, be followed by a corresponding quick drop due to the insulin response, and then you'll be on a sugar-craving roller coaster for the rest of the day. You can avoid this effect at most meals by including a healthy mix of all three macronutrients: protein, carbs, and fat. At each meal, if you eat the right amount of protein, the right amount of carbohydrates, the right amount of fat, and you make sure that your foods are nutrient dense, you'll do just fine.

Basically, there are two effective ways to ensure that you are meeting your protein needs.

1. For those who don't like math and like to keep things simple . . . Eat a portion of protein at each meal that is equal to the size of your palm. This is an effective and widely used method for its simplicity and accuracy. It's likely that our palm size corresponds closely to our overall size, whether we are big or small. For an average-sized adult, a palm-sized portion of animal protein provides about 30 grams of protein.

2. And for those who don't mind a little math . . . You can calculate your minimum daily protein needs. To do so, take your ideal body weight in pounds and multiply that by .5. That is, roughly, the *minimum* amount of grams of protein you should strive to eat every day. Divide that number by the number of meals you eat in a day to calculate your protein needs for each meal.

As an example, suppose your ideal weight is 150 pounds. Multiply that by .5, and you need a minimum of 75 grams of protein per day. Suppose you eat three meals per day. That's 25 grams per meal. If at that level you feel strong and your musculature is satisfactory, you can remain there. But if you don't feel strong at that level, or you are involved in strenuous work or sports, you may need to up the multiplier to .6 or .7, or even higher. Your body will let you know by how you feel. And when you become older, starting at about age 65, your percentage of protein should slightly increase.

Whether you use method one or two above, be flexible, according to your protein hunger. If you find yourself needing or craving a little more protein, or a little less, don't be afraid to adjust up or down according to your needs. Your body, when its signals are in tune and true, is quite the helpful guide.

You might ask, though, if there is any harm in overshooting our protein needs, just to make sure that we have enough. And that's a great question. Overconsuming protein can have potentially serious consequences. Excessive protein raises our blood levels of IGF-1

(Insulin-like Growth Factor-1). High levels of this hormone can make for some stupendous muscles, but it also raises our risk for cancer and other health maladies. Excessively high protein intake and the resultant rise in IGF-1 can feed and extend the life in cancer cells, which can keep them living and growing. In their book, *Eat Like the Animals*, Raubenheimer and Simpson write that "eating too much protein switches on biological processes that hasten aging and shorten lives." Elevated IGF-1 levels is one of those processes. So again, it's best to eat the amount of protein you need and not much more.

Should You Favor Plant or Animal Protein?

Should you favor plant or animal protein? This is, of course, a highly individual and sometimes deeply personal choice. You may decide to get all of your protein from plant-based foods. But it is generally recognized that animal proteins have a higher rate of digestibility and therefore are superior at building and maintaining muscle mass. For instance, there are indexes, or charts, that rate the availability to our bodies of various sources of protein. Perhaps the best scale is called the DIAAS (Digestible Indispensable Amino Acid Score).

On this scale, and other scales, animal proteins consistently and significantly outscore plant proteins for digestibility and availability. Animal proteins score very high, beans score somewhat lower, and grains score even lower. So, gram for gram of protein, animal proteins will be better used by our body to build and maintain muscle mass and strength.—See DIAAS Score Chart Below

DIAAS scores are classified as follows:
100+........................Excellent sources of protein
75-99 ....Good
Below 75 ....Suboptimal

Food	DIAAS Score
Whole Milk	114
Eggs (Hard Boiled)	113
Beef	111
Chicken Breast	108
Tilapia	100
Canned Tuna	100
Garbanzo Beans	83
Kidney Beans	59
Peas, Cooked	58
Oats	57
Peanuts	43
Wheat	40
Almonds	40
Corn	36

Again, it's understandable that many may have personal reasons for wanting to eat a fully plant-based diet. Many top nutritional experts, though, recommend a combination of both plant and animal-based proteins, focusing primarily on plant protein.

The Elderly and Protein

While we are discussing elevated IGF-1 and the increased risk of cancer, please note that nutritional scientists feel safe recommending higher protein intake for the elderly, and particularly those over 65. Here's why: As we age, IGF-1 levels gradually decline, and by the time someone reaches 65, he or she can eat a substantially increased amount of protein, and their IGF-1 levels will still remain relatively low. This gives them, if you will, immunity to many of the negative effects of eating too much protein. That, coupled with the resultant loss of muscle mass for those in that age group, makes it smart to increase, at least moderately, protein intake, including perhaps, high-quality animal proteins. The increased amount of protein, preferably along with some resistance strength training exercises, such as weightlifting, isometrics, or exercise bands, should yield good results.

Popular longevity expert Peter Attia (who looks amazing at 50+ years old) explains it this way: "In humans, low protein in the elderly leads to low muscle mass, yielding mortality and worse quality of life." No, we don't want that. So again, when someone reaches or approaches about age 65, they are wise to begin increasing their protein intake moderately. Longevity research expert Valter Longo explains: "Over age 65, you should slightly increase protein intake but also increase consumption of fish, eggs, white meat, and products derived from goats and sheep to preserve muscle mass. Consume beans, chickpeas, green peas, and other legumes as your main source of protein."

Others Who Made Need Additional Protein

Beside the elderly and those who need additional muscle strength to compete in sports or to work at manual labor, there are others who could benefit from a higher protein diet. These include those who are trying to lose weight, those with blood sugar or metabolic problems, the chronically ill, and those who are under a lot of stress.

According to functional medicine specialist Chris Kresser, those who are under great amounts of stress would benefit from including in their diets some proteins that are high in collagen, as collagen protein is used by our bodies at a higher rate when we are under a lot of stress. High collagen protein foods include bone broth, fish, chicken, organ meats, eggs (particularly the whites), and some plant food sources, including berries and broccoli. You can also use collagen protein powders.

Protein Leveraging

Please note one more fascinating aspect of dietary protein: We are wired, or programmed, to continue eating until our protein needs have been met. In other words, let's say you require 90 grams of dietary protein a day, or an average of 30 grams per meal. And suppose you sit down to a meal and load your plate with potatoes, bread, butter, olive oil, non-starchy veggies, and fruit. Will you be satisfied and satiated? Not likely. With those food choices, you may be consuming only about five to ten grams of protein during that meal. Your body knows that you need more, so you will likely continue to eat, and therefore overeat on carbs and fat in your attempt to get more protein in your body. (The foods in this example are mostly carbs and fat, but they do contain small amounts of protein.) And you can see where that is going to get you: Extra carbs, extra fat, extra calories, equals extra you, and in all the wrong places.

So, when planning your meals, it's a good idea to prioritize making sure that each meal contains the amount of protein that you need. That's known as protein leveraging. Those who leverage, or prioritize protein, find themselves satisfied with fewer calories in their diets and are therefore rewarded with trimmer, healthier bodies.

Note: This is not to say that we should all be eating high-protein diets. We've already established that it's best to eat as much protein as our bodies need and not much more. Rather, you practice protein leveraging by simply making sure that you are meeting your protein requirement at every meal. It's usually best to eat your higher protein foods earlier in the meal, which will help ensure that you are correctly practicing protein leveraging, which will prevent you from overeating carbs and fat.

Protein Powders

Finally, you may be wondering about using protein powders. That can be a good idea, especially if you are on a vegan diet or otherwise require additional protein. Many brands contain about 20 to 30 grams of protein per serving. But please do not become dependent on protein powders as your main source of protein. Rather, view protein powder as a supplement. It's preferable that a majority of your dietary protein comes from foods. Usually, a limit of one serving of protein powder daily is recommended.

The Recommended Healthy Approach for Protein

Adequate protein is essential to your muscle maintenance and overall health. It's best to make sure you are getting adequate protein for your needs but to not overindulge, which could present serious problems if done on a regular basis.

One of the easiest ways to ensure you are eating adequate protein is to eat a palm-sized portion of protein at each meal.

A second way, for those who don't mind math, is to calculate your minimum daily protein needs. To do so, take your ideal body weight in pounds and multiply that by .5. That is, roughly, the *minimum* amount of grams of protein you should strive to eat every day. Divide that number by the number of meals you eat in a day to calculate your protein needs for each meal. If you are involved in strenuous work or sports, you may need to up the multiplier to .6 grams, or .7, or even higher.

Whichever method you use, pay attention to how you feel. Be flexible. If you find yourself needing or craving a little more protein, or a little less, don't be afraid to adjust up or down according to your needs.

Animal protein is generally considered more potent at building muscles than plant protein, but it is still the course of wisdom to get most of our protein from plant sources. Some have found it helpful to include animal protein with one meal a day and to focus on plant protein at the others.

As we age, and especially after the age of 65, our ability to utilize protein decreases, so we need more protein in our diets. Those who are trying to lose weight, those with blood sugar or metabolic problems, the chronically ill, and those who are under a lot of stress may also need additional protein.

You can supplement your protein needs with protein powder. But be sure to use powders as a supplement and not as your main source of protein. Most of your protein intake should come from the foods you eat.

By practicing protein leveraging, that is, making sure that your protein needs are met each day and at each meal, you do your body a huge favor and will be rewarded with a more vibrant health outcome!

Chapter 3

Carbohydrates

● How many carbs should you be eating on a daily basis for optimal health? Very low, low, medium, or high amounts? Which carbs are the healthiest? What are slow carbs? How can the glycemic index and glycemic load help? Which carbs should be avoided?

Carbohydrates are a source of great controversy in the dietary world. Thankfully, virtually all responsible nutritional advisers recommend that we avoid refined carbs, such as sugar and flour. Where the controversy comes in, usually, involves the amount of carbs in our diets. Some recommend very low carb diets, such as the keto diet, with as little as 20 grams of carbs daily—which is so little that it's almost nothing. Others, especially those who recommend vegan diets, suggest that the world's healthiest people eat mainly carbohydrate diets, as high as 75 to 90 percent, which is hundreds of grams of carbs daily. That's a huge variation. Who is correct? We'll get to that in a moment.

What Do Carbohydrates Do, and Why Do We Need Them in Our Diets?

For many, and particularly those with a "sweet tooth," carbs are their absolute favorite. Of the three macronutrients, carbohydrates provide the quickest source of available energy to our bodies. And therein lies the main problem involving carbs—some forms of carbohydrates act much too quickly in the body, rapidly raising blood sugar, therefore spiking insulin, and thereby creating a host of problems, including unwanted weight gain. NOTE: Many believe that dietary fat causes weight gain. But dietary fat, and especially good fats, such as omega-3s and monounsaturated fats, are necessary for sound health, and they do not contribute to obesity when eaten in moderate amounts. It's excess carbs, and especially refined carbs, such as flour and sugar, that are most responsible for unwanted weight gain.

There are three main types of carbohydrates: sugars, starches, and fibers. Then there are many subtypes of each. For instance, it is now claimed that there are 61 types of sugar, including dextrose, fructose, glucose, lactose, maltose, sucrose, high-fructose corn syrup, and so on. Fiber is generally divided into two categories: soluble fiber and insoluble fiber, and while they are both beneficial, each acts differently in the digestive system. Gastroenterologist and gut and microbiome expert Will Bulsiewicz claims that the makeup of fiber in each plant is unique, and thus each has a unique effect on the body.

Slow Carbs Are the Best Carbs

For most of us, eating carbohydrates is not a problem. They are found abundantly in natural foods—in fact, in the plant kingdom, carbohydrates are the most abundant of the three macronutrients. Like everything else, we want to eat them in balance, so it's best to not let carbs overwhelm our diets. And when eating carbs, it's best to focus on those that are considered "slow carbs," which are those that do not raise your blood glucose levels excessively fast or to high levels. Carbs that digest slowly, thereby gently raising blood sugar levels, are much healthier.

What are fast carbs? Basically, they're the highly refined sugars and flours. An outstandingly clear example of this is soda. A typical 12-ounce can of cola contains about 40 grams of carbs, all of which are sugar. Cola has zero grams of protein, zero grams of fat, and zero fiber. So those 40 grams of sugar, which is the equivalent of about ten teaspoons of sugar, will enter your system rapidly, with no protein, fats, or fiber to slow down their absorption and the subsequent rapid rise in blood glucose. Thankfully, the added phosphoric acid and caffeine help to keep the sugars and your energy in a healthy balance. (Uh, kidding!)

Interesting Fact: Guess how much sugar is in the average adult human bloodstream. You may be surprised at the amount. The answer: About four grams of sugar, which is just about one teaspoon. That's right, just one teaspoon. So, you can see the problem when you suddenly dump ten teaspoons of sugar into your body. If all ten teaspoons were quickly assimilated and turned into blood sugar, your glucose level would be about 1,100 mg/dl (61.1 mmol/L). That would present a HUGE problem, to say the least. To prevent this, your body needs to quickly release large amounts of insulin, which lowers your blood sugar to safer levels. But excessive insulin in the blood brings some serious consequences. It's this very mechanism that has wreaked so much havoc in so many people.

Which foods qualify as slow carbs? These include such foods as non-starchy vegetables, minimally processed whole grains, and legumes. They digest slowly, thereby releasing sugar slowly, because they contain other nutrients that slow down processing, such as proteins, fats, and fiber. Fruits are generally considered to be moderate carbs. When you think of an apple, for instance, there's a little protein and a lot of fiber to slow the glycemic reaction. Sweeter fruits, though, such as certain melons, dates, overripe bananas, and dried fruits are almost pure sugar; these can raise your blood sugar more rapidly. So even with fruits, restraint is necessary.

Along those lines, many who are insulin sensitive, such as those who are diabetic or prediabetic, can still get quite a sugar rise from slow carb foods. They would need to be judicious in their consumption of all carbs. For instance, Mark Hyman, in his book *The Pegan Diet*, recommends that those with diabetes, prediabetes, or those struggling with their weight, limit starchy vegetables to just half a cup up to three times a week. They also do well to limit fruits to one or two servings per day, focusing on fruits that are lower in sugar, such as berries.

In general, it's best that your blood sugar levels don't rise more than about 30 mg/dl (1.7 mmol/L) after meals or snacks. (As measured one to two hours after eating.) Excess of that starts most people on a sugar roller coaster, with damaging effects to their health. One of the best ways to monitor this is by using a glucometer, which allows you to test your blood sugar levels instantly at home. Typical glucometers cost less than $35 US, and some of the cheaper ones do a solid and reliable job. Continuous glucose monitors are becoming more available and popular for those who need them.

Again, it's healthier when our blood sugar levels rise gently after meals, and the way to accomplish that is to make sure a majority of the carbs you eat are slow carbs, which release sugars into the bloodstream slowly and evenly.

The Glycemic Index and Glycemic Load

Two tools to help you choose carbs that are primarily slow carbs are the glycemic index and the glycemic load.

The *glycemic index* measures how fast various foods can make your blood sugar rise. The glycemic index grades foods on a scale of 1 to 100. Pure glucose has a glycemic index score of 100.

Glycemic Index scores are classified as follows:
0-55 ....Low Glycemic
56-69 ....Medium Glycemic
70-100 ....High Glycemic

Below is a list of some glycemic index scores: (If you need them, you can find more comprehensive listings on the Web.)

Glycemic <u>Index</u> Scores	
Food	**Score**
Fruit	
Lemon	21
Strawberries	25
Apple	38
Orange	42
Cantaloupe	63
Pineapple	65
Watermelon	72
Vegetables	

Olive Oil	0
Broccoli	6
Tomatoes	6
Brussels Sprouts	15
Carrots	47
Peas	48
Sweet Potato	61
French Fries	75
Baked Potato	85
Grains	
All Bran	42
Whole Grain Bread	51
Rice, Brown	55
Oatmeal	58
Rice, White	64
Bagel	72
White Bread	73
Cream of Wheat	74
Corn Flakes	81
Legumes	
Soybeans	16
Kidney Beans	24
Garbanzo Beans	28
Black Beans	30
Navy Beans	31
Lentils	32

Pinto Beans	33
Misc.	
Peanuts	14
Cashews	22
Snickers Bar	55
Corn Chips	63
Graham Crackers	74
Vanilla Wafers	77
Popcorn, plain	79
Pretzels	83
Glucose	100

The *glycemic load* is similar to the glycemic index, but it goes a step further. The glycemic load takes into account not only the glycemic index, but it also factors in the size of the typical serving of that food. Therefore, the glycemic load is considered more accurate and reliable, a better guide to accessing real-life situations. (That said, please note that it's my observation that people tend to refer to the glycemic index scale more than they do the glycemic load scale. And I get it. I find the glycemic load scale kind of awkward and clunky.)

Glycemic Load scores are classified as follows:
0-10 ....Low Glycemic
11-19 ....Medium Glycemic
≥ 20.........................High Glycemic

Below is a list of some glycemic load scores: (If you need them, you can find more comprehensive listings on the Web.)

Glycemic **Load** Scores		
Food	**Serving Size**	**Score**
Beef, Chicken, Fish	-----	0
Tomatoes	1 cup	1
Cabbage	1 cup	1
Broccoli	Half cup	1
Asparagus	6 spears	1
Cashews	1 ounce	2
Carrots, raw	1 cup	3
Lentils	1 cup	7
Kidney Beans	1 cup	8
Orange	1 medium	11
Orange Juice	8 ounces	13
Banana	1 whole	14
Pepsi	8 ounces	15
Corn on the Cob	1 ear	15
Apple	1 medium	15
Oatmeal	1 cup	16
French Fries	Half cup	22
Pasta	1 cup	25
Baked Potato	1 medium	33
Rice, White, Boiled	1 cup	35
Pancake	1 medium	39
Raisins	100 grams	46

Watermelon is sometimes used as an example of a food that has a high glycemic index score but a low glycemic load score. That is because watermelon is very sweet, mostly pure sugar and water, but the typical serving eaten is not very large. Therefore, a slice of watermelon won't have a drastic effect on blood sugar levels. Watermelon has a glycemic index of about 72 (high), but the glycemic load of a slice is only 5 (low). However, if you eat four servings at one time, the glycemic load then multiplies from 5 to 20, or from the low range to the high range. (Often, it's not only what we eat, but how much of it, that determines if that food will be healthful for us.)

The way foods are cooked can also have an effect on the glycemic index and glycemic load scales. For instance, pasta that is cooked al dente will digest more slowly than overcooked pasta. Therefore, al dente will not raise the blood sugar as quickly, giving it lower scores on both the glycemic index and glycemic load scales.

And sometimes other factors affect the scores. For instance, do you think that bananas are low on the glycemic index, medium glycemic, or high glycemic? The answer is, all three. Huh? Bananas that have sufficient green on the skins are considered low glycemic, yellow bananas are medium glycemic, and brown or spotted bananas are high glycemic. As bananas ripen, the sugar content increases dramatically.

Interesting Note: Which of the following foods would you consider to be a health food: a glazed donut, or a bagel? The answer: Neither, and neither one is close.

A glazed donut has 260 calories, 31 grams of carbs, and a glycemic load of 17.

A bagel has 290 calories, 56 grams of carbs, and a glycemic load of 33.

This comparison amazes most people, who just assume that the donut is worse. But the glycemic load of the bagel is essentially double that of the donut. While the donut has more sugar and tastes sweeter, the bagel is loaded with starch. That starch, especially in its flour form, will raise your blood sugar very quickly, and the sugar load on the body is substantial. For some reason, bagels are sometimes thought of as a health food. As you can see, they are not.

Author's note: But if you have to have an occasional bagel, you can dramatically blunt the glycemic response. How? Start by eating only half of the bagel, which will drop the glycemic load from 33 to 16.5. Then, if you add a little cream cheese, some lox, a slice of a ripe tomato, some onions, some capers, and perhaps some whitefish spread and olives, those additional foods, by contributing protein, fat, and some fiber, will slow the subsequent rise in your blood sugar.

(I haven't had a bagel in years, but by describing that as I just did, I practically talked myself into getting one. But better yet, rather than applying this principle with a bagel, do it with healthy, whole-grain foods, such as steel cut oatmeal. By adding olive oil, protein powder, nut milk, and flax or chia seeds, you will stunt the glycemic effect.)

Fiber

While fiber is a form of carbohydrate, it's not what we usually think of when we think of carbs. We tend to think of carbs as sources of quick energy. Fiber, on the other hand, provides almost no energy, as it remains largely undigested, and it actually serves to slow down the energy that is released in the body when we eat fiber along with such carbs as sugar and starches.

There are two main types of fiber: soluble fiber and insoluble fiber. Both are beneficial to our health. Soluble fiber is so named because it dissolves in water; insoluble fiber does not dissolve in water. Fiber is found only in plant products. (One reason I recommend NOT going on the "Carnivore diet.") Most plants contain a mixture of soluble fiber and insoluble fiber. By focusing on plant-based foods and eating a variety of them, you will be getting a nice mixture and an abundant amount of fiber in your diet.

Notice some of the health benefits from eating an abundance of fiber:

- Cholesterol level control
- Microbiome vitality
- Blood sugar control

- Better digestion
- Cancer prevention
- Better skin tone
- Better heart health
- Better mental clarity
- Increased meal satiation and satisfaction
- Weight loss

How much dietary fiber should you be eating on a daily basis? The USDA (United States Department of Agriculture) recommends that men eat 38 grams of fiber a day and that women eat 25 grams of fiber a day. Older men and women can slightly reduce that number. The bad news is that American adults eat a paltry 15 grams of fiber per day. That's about half of the daily recommendation. And in the opinion of many gut-health experts, the USDA's recommendations are too low. For most, it would definitely be a good idea to increase their consumption of fiber-rich plant-based foods.

There are many fiber supplements on the market, which are sold under many names. Some of the more popular ones are psyllium, acacia gum, inulin, wheat dextrin, and guar gum. These supplements can be helpful in raising your fiber intake. However, it's recommended that you get the bulk of your dietary fiber, not from supplements, but from plant-based foods.

Finally, while it's good to up your fiber intake, it's best to do so gradually, which will allow your body to adjust to the change. Too much fiber too soon can actually cause constipation. Furthermore, as you increase your fiber intake, you'll need to drink additional water. By eating according to the principles that will be outlined in this book, your fiber consumption will automatically reach healthy levels.

Net Carbs vs. Total Carbs

From time to time, you'll hear the terms "total carbs" and "net carbs." What's the difference?

"Total carbs" are just that, the total amount of carbohydrates in a food item from all sources, including sugars, starches, fibers, sugar alcohols, and so on. "Net carbs" are the total carbs minus fiber and sugar alcohols. This is because fiber and sugar alcohols are not processed in the body the way that sugars and starches are. Fiber is largely not digested and does not get converted to blood sugar. Sugar alcohols, such as xylitol and erythritol, taste very sweet, but they do not significantly raise blood sugar levels.

Let's take a look at a food label and see this in practice . . . Notice the label of a can of Organic Black Beans from Whole Foods. There are, per serving, 20 grams of carbohydrates, and there are 9 grams of fiber. So, doing the quick math (20 grams total carbs − 9 grams of fiber = 11 grams of net carbs), the net carbs per serving of these beans is 11.

Nutrition Facts

about 3.5 servings per container

Serving size   1/2 cup (130g)

Amount per serving

Calories 110

	% Daily Value*
Total Fat 0g	0%
Saturated Fat 0g	0%
Trans Fat 0g	
Cholesterol 0mg	0%
Sodium 85mg	4%
Total Carbohydrate 20g	7%
Dietary Fiber 9g	32%
Total Sugars <1g	
Includes 0g Added Sugars	0%
Protein 7g	

If you are concerned about your carbohydrate intake because of your glucose levels or weight issues, read the labels and do the math. Your focus should be on net carbs, not total carbs. Again, fiber does not raise blood sugar levels and actually helps to keep them lower. Fiber is the good guy!

Resistant Starch

Resistant starch has only recently become known and written about, and it's still somewhat of a "secret." What is resistant starch, and what does it do?

In the strictest sense of the term, it's starch that is resistant to something, and the good news is, that something just happens to be digestion—resistant starch is resistant to digestion. This means that foods with resistant starch will not raise blood glucose levels as much as those with regular starch. Resistant starch acts more like fiber in the body than it does starch. Therefore, because it is not fully digested, it also acts in the gut like a prebiotic, aiding microbiome health by feeding gut bacteria.

Which foods contain resistant starch? Some of the best-known sources are bananas with green skins (the banana skins don't have to be completely green, but the more green the skins, the more resistant starch in the fruit), potatoes (to maximize the resistant starch in potatoes, cook them and allow them to cool, then eat them—it's okay to reheat, which will not destroy the resistant starch), rice (also cooked and cooled), beans, lentils, yams, barley, cashews, and oats.

You can also buy resistant starch powders, usually made from potato starch or green banana starch. Dr. Mark Hyman is a big advocate for potato starch, which has only a minimal effect on blood sugar levels.

The Recommended Healthy Approach for Carbohydrates

Again, thankfully, all responsible nutritionists recommend that we avoid refined carbohydrates, such as sugar and flour. No controversy there. And just by taking that one step, that is, eliminating sugar and flour, you'll be improving your health significantly. Further, the vast majority consider non-starchy vegetables to be safe to eat in unlimited quantities. (Did you know that there are some vegetables that you could eat 24/7 and actually lose weight? For instance, it's believed that celery is a negative caloric food. In other words, it takes more calories for your body to digest and assimilate the celery you eat than is actually in the celery itself. By eating celery continually, you'll lose weight.)

So, we know that refined carbs are bad, and non-starchy vegetables are good. Therefore, the real question mark with carbohydrates involves those found in such foods as grains, beans, fruits, starchy vegetables, and maybe dairy (the middle zone on the chart). How much should we include in our diets? Is it better to aim for low amounts, high amounts, or somewhere in between?

Non-Starchy Vegetables	Eat Unlimited Amounts
The Carb Decision Zone **Starchy Vegetables** **Fruit** **Grains** **Legumes** **(Maybe) Dairy**	Eat According to Your Needs, Considering Your Weight, Level of Activity, and Metabolic Health
Refined Carbs (Sugar and Flour)	Avoid

Ideally, my blanket answer for all the macronutrients is moderate: moderate proteins, moderate carbohydrates, and moderate fats. In a perfect world, that is a perfect answer. But the world is not perfect, and our bodies are certainly not perfect. So, really, as with most areas in nutrition, the answer depends upon your needs and goals.

For those who have good metabolic health, generally meaning those who are not overweight and who have healthy glucose levels, moderate carbs, or about 40 to 50 percent of dietary calories, is a good amount. For those who are very active and who burn lots of calories and need additional fuel, some additional carbs should be well tolerated. (Also, it should be noted, many long-lived residents of the Blue Zones tend to eat a higher percentage of carbohydrate foods . . . perhaps 50 to 75 percent of their diets are carbohydrates, predominantly slow carbohydrates.)

But for those who have metabolic issues, which would include those with excess body fat and those who have elevated glucose levels, including those who are diabetic or are prediabetic (prediabetes is defined as fasting glucose levels between 100 mg/dl (5.6 mmol/L) and 125 mg/dl (6.9 mmol/L) or an (Hb) A1c reading between 5.7 and 6.4), reducing carbohydrate intake makes good sense. It's not that you have to go keto, but be careful to keep your carbohydrate intake on the low side, perhaps to less than 100 grams of net carbohydrates a day, depending on the severity of your condition. Ideally, it's best to eat only as many carbs as can be tolerated without raising your glucose levels by more than about 30 mg/dl (1.7 mmol/L) at any meal or snack. (Measured one to two hours after the meal.) And no matter what your metabolic health is, keep refined carbs to a strict minimum.

You do well to eat plenty of non-starchy vegetables, such as broccoli, greens, lettuces, peppers, zucchini, yellow squash, mushrooms, etc., at two or even all three of your meals each day. Dietician and author Chef AJ coined the acronym VFB, which stands for Vegetables For Breakfast. It may not be a standard eating practice, but it's a reasonable and healthful practice if you choose to incorporate it.

Eat non-starchy vegetables at most meals, eat moderate amounts of proteins with every meal, eat a serving of high-quality fats with each meal, and then eat, according to your energy needs, healthy slow-to-moderate carbs, such as legumes, minimally processed grains, fruits, starchy vegetables, and so on. By eating the carbohydrate-rich food toward the end of the meal, after you've eaten a good amount of protein and fiber, you will be further slowing your body's glycemic response to the carbs.

Carbs are wonderful, and they are found abundantly in nature. Eat them wisely, according to your body's needs, and focus on slow carbs, which are those that won't raise your blood sugar quickly. If you do this, your body will repay you with many benefits, including better weight control and more energy.

Chapter 4

Fats

• Is dietary fat healthy or is it damaging? Will it cause me to gain adipose tissue (bodily fat)? How much fat should I be eating on a daily basis for optimal health? Ultra-low, low, high, or somewhere in between? Are some fats better than others? Are fats heart-healthy? Do I need to include fats with every meal?

Lions and tigers and bears and dietary fat . . . oh my! Dietary fat is often vilified as a deadly killer, lurking in our food supply, just waiting to do us much bodily harm, proceeding straight from our mouths to our bellies, hips, and hindquarters, making us fat, and marching right into our arteries, clogging them, triggering heart attacks and strokes. And some of the world's top nutritionists, especially those who champion extreme low-fat diets, teach exactly that.

On the other hand, there is a growing number of nutritional experts who believe that a moderate and even abundant amount of dietary fat is an important part of a healthy diet. The range of recommended fat intake among nutritional experts is huge. Some suggest that we eat a maximum of ten percent fat (by calorie count) in our diets—I've even seen as low as eight percent. Many suggest a more moderate amount, such as 25-35 percent. Others, including most keto advocates, suggest really loading up on dietary fat, making it the prominent part of our diets, at about 75-80 percent. Again, that's a huge range. Your life is at stake. Who's right?

Some of the confusion with fat has to do with the English language itself. As Dr. Mark Hyman explains: "When it comes to fat, we have a semantics problem. In other languages, the word for the fat we eat is different from the word for the unwanted stuff clinging to our midsections."

Many words have double meanings, and some of those include words that are food related, such as "date." We can eat a date, and we can go on a date. No one would confuse the two. But dietary fat and bodily fat are just too close to not cause confusion.

Further, the various types of fat can be confusing. Some teach that there are good fats and bad fats. But it goes beyond that. There are essential fats, excellent fats, good fats, and terrible fats. Let's take a look at fat and sort things out.

What Do Fats Do, and Why Do We Need Them In Our Diets?

We technically need very little dietary fat in our diets to stay alive. But to be truly healthy, we need a more substantial amount. Note some of the reasons why, as explained by Mark Hyman in his groundbreaking book, *Eat Fat Get Thin*: "Eating more of the right fats helps you lose weight and prevent dementia, heart disease, diabetes, and cancer, all while giving you the added side benefits of improved mood, skin, hair, and nails." Then, speaking specifically of monounsaturated fats, he writes: "They improve insulin sensitivity and therefore reduce diabetes risk, reduce breast cancer risk, reduce pain in people with rheumatoid arthritis, promote weight loss, and reduce belly fat." That's quite a list of positives, and clearly, we want to enjoy those benefits if possible.

Energy Density

Fats are the most calorically dense nutrient. While the other two macronutrients, protein and carbohydrates, yield four calories per gram, a gram of fat yields nine calories. Fats do not build muscle tissue, protein does that. And fats do not provide much instant energy, carbs do that. But fats are satiating, and they provide the body with stability as they help with many bodily functions.

Types of Fat

Essential fatty acids are those that cannot be made in the human body. This includes omega-3 fats Eicosapentaenoic acid (EPA), Docosahexaenoic acid (DHA), and Alpha-linolenic acid (ALA). EPA and DHA are derived from seafood, and ALA is found in a variety of foods, including walnuts, flax seeds, chia seeds, and some leafy vegetables and animal fats.

In addition to the essential fatty acids, there are four general classes of dietary fats. They are Saturated Fat, Unsaturated Fat (including Monounsaturated and Polyunsaturated Fats), and Trans Fat. Each of these fats has a unique chemical structure and a different effect on the body.

Saturated fats are often referred to as "bad fats." That is somewhat of a misnomer. Because saturated fats tend to raise cholesterol levels, it may be beneficial to limit them in our diets and to favor unsaturated fats. But limit and shun are not the same, and there is no reason to shun saturated fats. They are a normal part of a healthy diet. Saturated fats are usually associated with meat and dairy, but they are found, to a degree, in many other foods that even vegans consider to be healthful, such as grains, fruits, and vegetables. Coconuts are loaded with saturated fat; even a bowl of oatmeal has a moderate amount of saturated fat. So does olive oil.

Monounsaturated and polyunsaturated fats both play key roles in a healthy diet. Omega-3s, described earlier as an essential fatty acid, are considered polyunsaturated fats. Olive oil, as well as avocados, are rich in monounsaturated fats. Research shows that replacing some saturated fat with mono and polyunsaturated fat tends to lower blood cholesterol.

Then there is trans-fat. (You can start booing now.) Yes, trans fats are really, really bad for you—in fact, they are deadly. They are found in highly processed foods, such as pies, cakes, and pastries . . . as if the refined sugar and flour does not cause enough damage. They are also abundant in deep fried foods and highly processed fast foods. Hydrogenated fats, and even partially hydrogenated fats, also tend to be high in levels of trans fat. This type of fat is a known contributor to the development of coronary heart disease. If at all possible, avoid trans fats.

Dietary Fat Helps with Vitamin and Mineral Absorption

When eating vegetables, such as a big salad or plate of steamed vegetables, we would waste a lot of vitamins and minerals if we did not include some fat in our meal. But when fat is included, vitamin and mineral absorption is increased. This is one reason why it's recommended that each meal is balanced with a portion of protein, carbohydrates, and fat. This wholesome benefit is enhanced when the fat is from a healthful source, such as olive oil, avocados, or raw nuts and seeds.

How Did We Become So Dietary Fat Phobic?

What, exactly, happened to cause us to become so afraid of dietary fat? And how has this fear worked out: has it helped to improve our individual and collective health, or has it hurt it?

In many ways, it started with Dwight Eisenhower, who was the 34th president of the United States. In September 1955, President "Ike" suffered a heart attack while serving in office. Just a few years prior to this, heart attacks were relatively rare in the United States. The rate of deaths from heart disease more than doubled in the thirty years between 1920 and 1950. So, when the sitting president of the United States suffered a heart attack in 1955, at the relatively young age of 64, the matter had everyone's attention. Suddenly, heart disease was a pressing national (and soon to be global) concern.

At this same time, in the 1950s, scientist Ancel Keys began a large-scale study of the effects of saturated fats on heart disease. Keys was the force behind the famous Seven Countries Study, where he used data from seven countries to "prove" that dietary fat, and particularly saturated fat, leads to greater incidence of heart disease and heart attacks. He thus promoted what is called the "diet-heart hypothesis." Based on the study and the hypothesis, Keys strongly recommended that people lower their intake of all fats and especially saturated fats.

But there was a problem with his method of research, which has since been uncovered and written about by many. Perhaps the most notable among those has been science journalist Nina Teicholz. In her

New York Times bestselling book, *The Big Fat Surprise*, she discusses how, while Keys used data from seven countries in his Seven Countries Study, he discarded data that he collected from 15 other countries. Guess what the data from those 15 discarded countries all had in common? That's right . . . simply, the data from those countries did not match his conclusions.

Those countries, which comprised a majority of the countries under consideration, showed no relationship between fat and heart disease. In other words, Keys cherry-picked his data to match his conclusion. And in the world of science, that's never a good thing, nor is it ethical. And in the world of, well, real life, the results, especially involving a subject dealing with life and death, can be fatal. Many responsible scientists believe this is exactly what happened with Keys and his conclusions. That is, bad science led to fatal consequences.

Suddenly, the dietary climate in the United States was changing. In the 1970s, Senator George McGovern headed a governmental committee that studied the matter of heart health and nutrition. The results, called "The McGovern Report," published in 1977, suggested that Americans eat less fat, and especially less saturated fat, as well as less cholesterol. The committee also recommended such prudent steps as eating only as many calories as are necessary and consuming more complex carbohydrates and fiber.

But what happened? Starting shortly after the release of the report, heading into the 1980s, these ripples of change in the dietary climate began to widen. While the McGovern report recommended such positive changes as eating more complex carbohydrates and fiber and eating only the amount of calories that are needed for good health, those suggestions seemed to quickly fade to the background. Rather, the main focus landed on fat and saturated fat. We tend to focus more on what is bad than what is healthful, as fear is a very strong motivator. All of a sudden, dietary fat had become nutritional enemy number one.

It should not be surprising that commercial interests quickly took advantage of this new climate. Multi-billion-dollar companies saw the opportunity and seized it. For instance, Nabisco launched a very popular line of low-fat snack foods called SnackWells. They were quite the rage for a while, and admittedly, they tasted pretty good. (I'm not going beyond "pretty good," because they were never great . . . Looking back, "pretty good" might even be a stretch.) How did SnackWells succeed in making their foods palatable?

It's well known that there are certain food items that our taste buds find appealing. At the top of this list are sugar and fat. The sugar AND fat combination is especially alluring. But SnackWells and others had a little dilemma. How would they make very low-fat foods taste good? They did this by simply increasing the amount of sugar. To many, if not most, sugar, which acts like a drug in our bodies and to our brains, can be irresistible. People were willing to forego the fat for an extra hit of sugar, especially when they thought that by doing so, they were doing the right thing for their bodies.

This is not what McGovern's committee intended. Their findings actually cautioned against increased sugar intake; they recommended more complex carbs and fiber. But most of the findings of the McGovern report got lost in public perception. That perception became, simply, avoid fat as much as possible, and especially saturated fat, and you and your heart will thrive. And you can be sure that this public perception was fueled and solidified by the millions of dollars these food manufacturers spent through their advertising agencies. There's lots of money to be made by marketing processed products in shiny, colorful packages created by the best minds at the best advertising firms. But marketing complex carbs and fiber, such as lettuce and broccoli . . . not so much.

That's how the low-fat craze got started and grew. But the key question is, what has been the result? Remember, the switch to a low-fat diet was supposed to make us trim and fit and improve our cardiac health. Fascinatingly, the exact opposite happened: It was at this very time that obesity rates began to soar. This is clinically proven through much research and data.

If you were alive in the late 1970s and early 80s, likely your memory will verify this fact. And if you look at videos from the 1960s and 70s, you'll find that very few people were obese. Go back further to pictures and videos of the early 1900s, and you'll find that most people were trim and fit. The terms "obese" and "obesity" were rarely used just fifty years ago; now they are a very common part of our language. The sad term "morbidly obese" has had increased usage in recent years too—the condition was barely known before 1980.

Dietary fat was never the problem causing obesity. The biggest problem was actually a carbohydrate, namely, sugar. Large amounts of sugar affect us hormonally and in other ways that cause us to store bodily fat. Add in the abundance of hyper-processed foods, and the unnatural combining of refined carbohydrates and fats, especially bad fats, and the results are stunning. The health of the general public today is atrocious. But as you can see, sadly, a lot of it got started following the events involving the heart attack of President Eisenhower in 1955. Many involved were well meaning, but a combination of bad science and slick marketing spewed misinformation, and the results have been deadly.

Interestingly, the rate of deaths from heart attacks rose significantly during much of the 20th century. But dietary fat consumption stayed relatively level during that time and even decreased. But what of the rate of consumption of sugar? It rose significantly. This provides further evidence that it's not dietary fat that causes heart disease, but the main culprit, rather, is sugar.

The bottom line of all of this is don't be afraid of dietary fats in general, and don't be overly afraid of saturated fats unless your level of LDL is high. Eat these fats in moderation and be very wary of refined carbohydrates, which are the real heart assassins.

The Recommended Healthy Approach for Fats

Dietary fats are found in a wide variety of foods, and there is no evidence that a balanced intake of fat leads to heart issues, such as clogging of the arteries, heart attacks, and strokes. That view is shared by many nutritional experts whom I deeply admire, including Mark Hyman, Chris Kresser, Joel Fuhrman, cardiologist Stephen Sinatra, cardiologist Steven Gundry, nutritionist Lindsay Christensen, and a vast host of others. I agree with them; a moderate amount of the right fats is not only harmless, but it is beneficial to the health seeker. The right fats in the right amounts are known to actually decrease your risk of heart disease.

Include a serving of fat at each meal. A serving of fat can be a tablespoon or two of olive oil, half an avocado, an ounce or handful of nuts and seeds, or other similar foods. Aim for three to five servings of fat each day.

In general, I recommend that for most people, about 30 to 35 percent of our diets should be comprised of calories from fat. That's actually very close to what the average American is doing in 2024. However, while the amount is correct, there needs to be an adjustment in the type of fat being consumed. Americans, and others in most industrialized nations, tend to eat a lot of saturated and even trans-fat. When those fats are replaced by more healthful fats, such as omega-3s, monounsaturated fat, and polyunsaturated fat, good health outcomes usually follow.

The Various Food Types

Chapter 5

Vegetables

Parent and teenage child having a conversation on the telephone, while the parents are away for a week:

Mother: Since we've been away, have you eaten anything green?

Teen: Only the bread.

● Thankfully, there's not a lot of controversy involving vegetables. Everyone (almost) knows how good they are for us and how important they are to a balanced and healthy diet. And yet, there are still some who believe that vegetables aren't so important. Among those are adherents to the Carnivore Diet and those on the SAD (Standard American Diet). Sadly, only about 10 percent of the American public eats the 5 to 7 servings of fruit and vegetables per day that many reputable sources recommend. Some almost never eat vegetables. And what about French fries? Do they count as a vegetable?

In food pyramids of not so many years ago, grains often formed the base of those pyramids, meaning that they were considered to be the foundation, or the most important part, of a healthy diet. In recent years, pyramids, such as those by Mark Hyman, Mark Sisson, and Joel Fuhrman, have been produced with vegetables at the base of the pyramid. That's good news, because many functional medicine and nutritional specialists now consider vegetables, which are loaded with nutrients, to be the most beneficial part of our diet. Vegetable types include leafy greens (lettuce, spinach, etc.), cruciferous (kale, broccoli, cauliflower, Brussels sprouts, cabbage), allum (garlic, onions), edible plant stem (asparagus, celery), root (potatoes, sweet potatoes, turnips, carrots), and others. Each type of vegetable brings specific health benefits to the body. Most notably, perhaps, is that cruciferous vegetables are highly protective against cancer and heart disease, and allum vegetables are also highly protective against certain cancers, including those of the gastrointestinal tract. Leafy green vegetables are often considered to be the most nutritious food on the planet.

Eat the Rainbow

One of the catchiest health phrases in recent years is "eat the rainbow." And it is indeed a good idea. But what does it mean? Simply, it means to eat produce in all colors of the rainbow. And there is an abundance of food in all of the various colors, some of which are listed below:

Red: Cherries, Cranberries, Tomatoes, Strawberries, Watermelon

Orange: Apricot, Butternut Squash, Carrots, Mangos, Pumpkin, Peaches, and, of course, Oranges

Yellow: Bananas, Corn, Grapefruit, Lemon, Yellow Squash

Green: Asparagus, Avocado, Celery, Cucumbers, Mint, Lettuce, Kale, Peas

Blue: Blueberries, Blue Corn, Blackberries (which are actually very dark blue), Concord Grapes

Indigo: Boysenberries, Plums, Prunes

Violet: Cabbage, Eggplant, Lavender, Passionfruit

Why is it important to eat the rainbow? Of course, the variety itself adds beauty to our meals, but more importantly, each color tends to bring with it certain specific nutrients. For instance, orange produce is rich in beta carotene, potassium, lycopene, flavonoids, and vitamin C. These beneficial substances are known to help your heart health, immune system, eyes, and bones. They also protect you from cancer. Other colors provide their own specific benefits.

Interesting note: You can eat the rainbow with tomatoes alone, as there are tomato varieties in all colors of the rainbow. There are, in fact, over 10,000 different types of tomatoes. Potatoes come close to hitting the complete rainbow. There are over 2,000 varieties of potatoes. They are all healthy, but if you see a potato that has turned green, it's best to avoid it. That means it's been exposed to too much light, and a slightly toxic substance called solanine has been formed.

Which is Healthier, Cooked or Raw Veggies?

The answer may be surprising. Some people assume that raw vegetables are healthier than cooked. After all, raw means untouched, crisp, juicy, as fresh as can be. Some raw foodists refer to cooked vegetables as "dead food." Is it?

Not at all. Nutritional analysis shows that cooked foods (cooked, not "nuked" in a microwave), retain much of their nutritional properties. Some people, particularly those with digestive difficulties, may gain more benefit from eating cooked vegetables, as those tend to be easier to digest than raw. Especially would this be true with hard vegetables, such as broccoli. Many top nutritional experts recommend that you include both raw and cooked vegetables in your diet. That is an excellent option. And some find it beneficial to eat more cooked vegetables in the colder months and more raw vegetables in the warmer weather.

For most root vegetables, such as potatoes, sweet potatoes, yams, rutabagas, and the like, cooked is definitely preferred by most people.

The most healthful methods of cooking vegetables are steaming, boiling, baking, and roasting. Stir fry, in a small amount of healthful oil, such as avocado, olive, or coconut oil, works too. But what about deep frying vegetables? Read on.

Are French Fries Vegetables?

I'll answer this by means of an illustration. Have you ever driven by a junk yard and seen where cars have been crushed and smashed down and then stacked up together? This is done when the vehicle is no longer useful; it will now be sold for scrap metal. Technically, that smashed vehicle is still a car; it has not suddenly become a boat. But is it really still a car? In reality, it's lost all of the properties that make it a car—you can't drive it anymore.

It's the same with French fries. They are still at their core made from potatoes. They haven't morphed into, say, a dairy product. But they have lost all of the healthful qualities that made them a vegetable in the first place, and there's been lots of nasty stuff added to them.

Some still want to consider French fries to be a vegetable. And whether you do or not is your choice. But please, for your body's sake, don't include deep fried vegetables, including French fries, when you tally your daily servings of vegetables. Of course, better yet, don't include them in your diet at all. They are loaded with trans-fat and they are health wreckers.

How Many Servings Per Day?

Most reputable sources recommend that we consume a minimum of 4 to 5 servings of vegetables and fruit per day. Some break that down to about 3 servings of vegetables and 2 servings of fruit. Dr. Mark Hyman sets the bar really high for the number of vegetables we should eat. He writes: "While the minimum recommended amount of veggies is 5 to 9 servings (1/2 cup per serving), I recommend 6 to 8 cups of vegetables (or 12 to 18 servings). Try to include as much variety as possible." Eight cups equal half a gallon, so you can see that is an ambitious goal. Dr. Hyman's diet, while containing adequate amounts of protein and fats, is centered on vegetables, and that is an excellent way to eat.

Most Americans do not eat the recommended minimum of 4 to 5 servings, so if you do, you are doing relatively well. That said, try to increase your total up to six cups, or 12 servings, if you can. You don't have to hit that goal, but the closer you come, the better. Dr. Hyman mentioned the importance of eating a variety of vegetables, and that's important too. Some have faced ill effects from eating too much of one certain vegetable, such as spinach, which can easily happen if you eat a lot of smoothies. Many vegetables contain substances, called "anti-nutrients," that are healthy in moderate amounts but can become toxic in larger doses. (Examples of anti-nutrients are oxalates, phytic acid, and lectins.) It's better to mix it up and eat the rainbow.

Starchy vs. Non-starchy

Vegetables can be broken down into two groups: starchy and non-starchy. There are a few vegetables that straddle that line, such as carrots. I've seen carrots listed as both starchy and as non-starchy vegetables. One nutritionist put them in both categories: he considers raw carrots to be non-starchy and cooked carrots to be starchy.

Because of glycemic issues, it's important to understand which category the different vegetables fit in. Non-starchy vegetables are considered the safest and healthiest foods in the world by many, and they can usually be eaten in unlimited amounts. But starchy vegetables contain, well, starch, and starch can quickly raise your blood sugar. Especially if you have issues with blood sugar control, or even body weight, it's important to be judicious with how much starch you eat.

Most vegetables are non-starchy, and they include greens, celery, broccoli, cabbage, mushrooms, asparagus, zucchini, yellow squash, cauliflower, artichokes, eggplant, sprouts, etc. Non-starchy vegetables do not have a sweet taste.

Starchy vegetables include corn, potatoes, sweet potatoes, yams, turnips, green peas, beets, butternut squash, acorn squash, and cassava. Starchy vegetables have a sweet taste.

The Recommended Healthy Approach for Vegetables

Vegetables are a key to a healthy diet. Those who make vegetables the predominant part of their diets usually enjoy very good health outcomes. Two of my favorite health writers point this out. Dr. Joel Fuhrman sums this up well when he says: "Vegetables—both raw and cooked—at the bottom take up the most room on the pyramid, and these should be the foods you eat the most." Dr. Mark Hyman adds: "If the bulk of your diet comes from non-starchy veggies, you are setting yourself up for success."

I agree, veggies should be your number one target, and it's best to eat them both raw and cooked. Try to include a salad with green leafy vegetables every day. And make sure to eat the rainbow, getting a wide variety of colorful vegetables into your diet. Aim for 4 to 8 cups daily, or 8 to 16 servings. That's an ambitious goal. But if you eat only half that amount, you are doing well.

It's best to eat a little fat with your vegetables, which will help you absorb the nutrients in those veggies. A healthy fat, such as a tablespoon or so of olive oil, might be ideal. But you can sprinkle seeds or nuts and have the same effect.

Buy the best quality veggies you can afford—organic if possible.

Many of us heard from the time that we were little that we should eat our vegetables. Mom and dad and grandma and grandpa were right after all. Vegetables are widely considered the most healthful food on the planet.

Chapter 6

Fruits

● **Fruits are normally part of a healthy diet. But fruits can contain a lot of sugar. How much fruit should you eat in a day, and are certain fruits healthier than others?**

Do you like candy? Fruit has been called "nature's candy." And rightly so, because it's perhaps the closest natural food to candy on the planet. The variety of fruit is pretty astounding. Considering just apples alone, there are at least 7,500 different varieties. We are probably all familiar with the most popular ones: Gala, Fuji, Granny Smith, Honeycrisp, Red and Golden Delicious, Envy, Dog's Snout, McIntosh. My favorite is Pacific Rose, which reminds me of candy apples on a stick. (Did Dog's Snout catch your attention? I was kidding about it being a popular type of apple, but it really is an apple variety, although quite unknown. It's shaped like a dog's snout.)

Fruits, like vegetables, are loaded with nutrients. Many fruits are particularly high in vitamin C. There is, though, a need to be judicious about the amount of fruit we eat per day. Fruit tends to be high in sugar, and too much sugar, even natural sugar, has negative effects on our health.

You may not know that fruits have undergone a change in recent decades. Jessie Inchauspé explains this in her book *Glucose Revolution: The Life-Changing Power of Balancing Your Blood Sugar*: "The fruit we eat these days has been bred for centuries to contain more glucose and fructose and less fiber than before." Taste wise, that's a good thing. Health wise, not so much. But food manufacturers know what people want, and sugar it is, so sales will increase if the sugar content is higher. Sadly, so do blood glucose levels and resulting incidence of diabetes, heart disease, and other maladies that accompany high sugar intake.

Eat Fruits That Are in Season

This is referred to as "seasonal eating," and it's the course of wisdom to follow it to the extent possible. Why? For the same reason many, if they are visiting a location close to the sea, will try to have at least one meal at a seafood restaurant. They know that the fish will be fresher and will taste better and be more nutritious.

I like how the website Eat the 80 (eathe80.com) explains this: "Fresher, sweeter, better-tasting, more flavorful and vibrant fruits and vegetables are what you have to look forward to when you choose to eat with the seasons!" You can add to that more nutritious too! In season fruit is more likely to be grown on local soil. Fruit that is picked out of season endures long storage periods and is subjected to cooling and heating to control ripeness. Such fruit is lacking; really, it's a cheap imitation of local fresh-picked produce.

Which Fruits Are Preferable?

Which are the good fruits, and which are the bad fruits? Really, they are all good and are properly viewed as gifts. However, some fruits are preferable to others, depending on the situation and circumstances. The main issue is sugar. Some fruits contain moderate amounts of sugar, whereas others are very high in sugar. And because so many people struggle with glucose control issues, there is a need to be careful with the types of fruit and amounts eaten. Notice the lists below of some lower and higher sugar fruits. It's best to eat more of the low sugar fruits, especially if you are overweight or have glycemic control issues.

Low Sugar Fruits (List by Ariel Klein)
Citrus

Berries

Kiwi

Cantaloupe

Peaches

Avocado (Usually eaten as a vegetable, but it's a fruit)

Apricots

Figs

Cranberries

Pomegranates

High Sugar Fruits

Grapes

Cherries

Bananas (depending on the level of ripeness)

Dried Fruits

Mangoes

Persimmons

Dates

Many nutritional experts agree that berries are probably the safest fruit to eat on a regular basis. They are low glycemic and are packed with nutrients. Many successfully eat berries every day. Of course, berries have a relatively brief ripe season, but frozen berries are a good option. Those berries are picked ripe and frozen immediately, so they retain most of their nutrients. Frozen berries are a wonderful addition to smoothies.

Don't Eat Naked Fruits

Do you mean, don't peel my apple before I eat it? No, the practice of not eating naked fruits refers to not eating fruit alone, by itself. That is usually recommended because "naked fruit" tends to send blood sugar levels up quickly. By adding a handful of nuts or seeds, a spoon of nut butter, some protein or some extra fiber, you'll be slowing down the glycemic response and leveling out your blood sugar levels. This leads to better blood sugar control throughout the day and to many fine benefits, such as weight loss. And remember, the sweeter the fruit and the greater quantity you eat, the more important it is to refrain from eating that fruit alone.

How Much Fruit Should You Eat Per Day?

Again, this depends upon your circumstances, and especially your glycemic status. If you have no issues with blood sugar control, you can safely eat two or perhaps three servings of fruit per day. But if you are overweight or have blood sugar issues, it's best to limit your fruit intake to one or two servings per day and to focus on fruits that are known to be lower glycemic.

The Recommended Healthy Approach for Fruits

Fruits are a natural delight. They are delicious and nutritious, and they are rightly referred to as "nature's candy." It's good to include a variety of fruit in your diet. However, because of the high sugar content in fruit, it's important to be judicious with the amount of fruit you eat. Those who are at a healthy weight and do not have glycemic issues can safely eat two or three servings of fruit a day. Those who are overweight or have glycemic issues should limit their fruit intake to one or two servings a day. They should focus, primarily, on low-glycemic fruits, such as berries.

Fruits are a delight, so eat them slowly, chew well, and savor each bite!

Chapter 7

Beans, Legumes

● Beans run the full gamut from glowing respect to disdain in the field of modern nutrition. Those on the paleo diet, which has a substantial following, shun beans. Others, including those in the long-lived Blue Zones, thrive on beans, eating about a cup a day, which equals about ten percent of their daily caloric intake. Some even consider beans to be the perfect food. Who is correct? Are beans truly a health food, or do the "antinutrients" lectins and phytic acid make them a menace? Should you eat beans, and if so, how much? Are there any other suggestions regarding beans?

"Paleo dogma on legumes holds that we should avoid them because they contain toxic anti-nutrients called lectins and phytic acid (aka phytate)." Functional medicine specialist Chris Kresser

"Beans are considered a 'superfood' because they are one of the most nutritious foods you can eat." University of Massachusetts Chan Medical School

"[Beans] reign supreme in the Blue Zones and are the cornerstone of every longevity diet in the world." Dan Buettner, Blue Zones expert

Note: Legumes is the broad category that includes beans, lentils, and peas. Carob, peanuts, and soybeans are legumes too. In this chapter, I'll be focusing on beans and lentils.

Do lectins and phytic acid make beans undesirable? A case can be made, and has been made, that EVERY food has its drawbacks. Recently, even vegetables, which should form the bulk of the most healthful diets, have been under attack because they contain natural toxins. But, of course, we can't stop eating everything. The key is balance, wisdom, and good judgement.

Beans Have a Lot Going for Them

"Beans could be nature's perfect food. These little powerhouses are packed with vitamins, minerals and phytochemicals." Karen Ansel, M.S., RDN

Beans are nutritional powerhouses. They are loaded with fiber, and fiber feeds the microbiome and helps to slow the glycemic response. This serves as a weight reduction aid. Beans are relatively high in protein, which makes them especially important for those on vegan diets. They are also packed with nutrients, especially folate and minerals, including hard to get minerals like magnesium, zinc, and potassium. And here is a fact that is not well known: You even get a little shot of beneficial omega-3 fats with beans.

Even though beans do contain significant starch, they are still a relatively low glycemic food. Dr. Joel Fuhrman explains it this way: "Beans improve blood sugar, whether you have diabetes or not. Beans contain fiber and resistant starch, which behave differently than grains and other carbohydrate sources. Multiple clinical trials have demonstrated that beans, lentils, and split peas improve blood sugar control."

Resistant starch is a health wonder. But what is it resistant to? To digestion. Therefore, instead of breaking down rapidly like most starch, resistant starch breaks down slowly, and much of the resistant starch never gets digested at all. In turn, this undigested starch feeds your gut buddies, making your microbiome healthier. It's for this reason that beans, in moderate amounts, are often recommended for diabetic patients. It's also why beans provide what is known as "The Second Meal Effect." This means that beans have been shown to help with your blood sugar regulation the meal *after* you eat them, whether or not you eat beans again with that meal. It's also believed this phenomenon occurs with meals *the day after* you eat beans, whether or not you eat beans that day.

Beans are a Staple of Blue Zones Diets

Dan Buettner, discussing residents of the Blue Zones who have lived extraordinarily long lives, says: "I can tell you beyond a shadow of a doubt that they're eating about a cup of beans a day." He also writes: "People in the Blue Zones eat at least four times as many beans as Americans do on average." Dan Buettner is considered the top Blue Zones expert, and he has spent much time with residents in all five Blue Zones. He's even published a Blue Zones cookbook with many recipes that feature beans.

Limits on Bean Consumption?

But does this mean that everyone should eat beans and eat them in unlimited amounts? No. For those who do eat beans, it's best to limit them to about one-half to one cup a day. Additionally, some would do well to further restrict their bean intake. For instance, beans are known as a pretty good source of protein. And while that is true, it's also true that beans contain more carbohydrates than protein. In fact, using pinto beans as an example, there are three times as many carbohydrates in a serving of pinto beans than there is protein. Many people, and especially those who are diabetic and prediabetic, need to be careful with their carbohydrate intake, keeping it on the low side.

Those with digestive difficulties may need to be judicious with their consumption of beans. If you struggle with digestive issues but still want to include beans in your diet, you would do well to work them in gradually. Perhaps start with just a couple of ounces at a time and gradually increase if you find that you are tolerating them well. Your microbiome will likely adjust in time, and you will be able to tolerate higher amounts of beans.

How To Cook Beans

Give attention to how your beans are cooked. True, beans do contain the "anti-nutrients" lectins and phytic acid, but they can be reduced greatly in the cooking process. How? The first step is to soak the beans in water, preferably overnight or even longer, for up to 24 hours. Much of the lectins and phytates will be washed away in the soaking water. And, as lectin-hater Dr. Steven Gundry recommends, as do others, cook your beans in a pressure cooker, which further destroys the lectins and phytates. Also, make sure to never eat undercooked beans, especially kidney beans.

The Recommended Healthy Approach for Beans and Legumes

Beans are so nutritious and versatile that even some of those who have ties to the paleo diet allow room for bean consumption. Simply put, there is just too much going for beans to shun them from our diets: They are filled with many nutrients, they are versatile and form the basis of many delicious meals, and perhaps more so than any other food item, they are gentle on our budgets. Unless there is a reason that you can't eat beans, such as an allergy or you need to be on a very low carb diet, you can probably safely and happily eat ½ cup to one cup of beans every day. Many nutritionists often recommend lentils, but really any bean, properly soaked and cooked, can be a staple in our diets.

So that's about it for the chapter on beans. Short and sweet. I hope you are able to incorporate beans into your diet and enjoy and benefit from them on a regular basis.

Fun Fact: Two varieties of beans have names that are the same as horse names: pinto beans and appaloosa beans. The word pinto literally means "painted," and it implies white with patches of other colors, which is true of pinto beans and pinto horses. Appaloosa beans and horses both have spotted patterns. And finally, the fava or broad bean is sometimes called the "horse bean."

Chapter 8

Grains

• Grains are one of the most debated areas in nutrition. Just years ago, grains formed the base of food pyramids and were considered the number one staple food in the American diet. Many today are leery of grains, and some, including those on the Paleo diet, avoid them completely, viewing grain's gluten, lectins, and phytates as being harmful and unfit for consumption . . . Are grains okay to eat, and if so, how much should you include in your diet?

Among the nutritional experts, the consensus is . . . that there is no consensus regarding grains! Rather, their viewpoints are all over the map. Some of the best minds in the field advise starting your day with a bowl of oatmeal and continuing to eat grains throughout the day. This is especially true in the vegan arena, where food choices are already quite limited. Others view grains as a dangerous food, and grains are on their "do not eat" list. Still others fall somewhere in the middle.

Should grains be off limits because they contain the "antinutrients" gluten, lectins, and phytates? Not necessarily. But if you have a specific illness, such as gluten intolerance or celiac disease, then, of course, you should be intolerant of allowing yourself to eat what is clearly going to harm you. It's no trivial matter, as the Celiac Disease Foundation explains: "When people with celiac disease eat gluten (a protein found in wheat, rye, and barley), their body mounts an immune response that attacks the small intestine."

But for the general public, those without such a specific intolerance, please note that vegetables also contain antinutrients, such as lectins, oxalates, phytates, and tannins. If you took dietary advice to the extreme, you could easily be talked into eating nothing, because every food, even healthful ones, can have some type of drawback.

Grains Are a Medium-High Glycemic Food

Those with weight control and glycemic control problems also need to be careful with grain products. Grains are a high carb food, and they can raise blood sugar levels quickly.

Dr. Sarah Ballantyne, author of *Nutrivore: The Radical New Science for Getting the Nutrients You Need from the Food You Eat*, highlights this point: "Eating grains to get more fiber is like eating carrot cake to get more vegetables. There is far more sugar in whole grains than in vegetables and even fruits."

I love the way Dr. Mark Hyman sums up his recommendation for grain intake. He writes: "As with most foods, the dose of grains is key. I recommend ½ cup to 1 cup of grains per day. If you are an athlete and are metabolically healthy (only 12 percent of us), you may be able to include more grains."

If You Eat Grains, Eat Those That Are Minimally Processed

If you do eat grains, it's important to eat grains that are minimally processed. The more a grain, or any food, is processed, the more nutrients it loses and the higher glycemic it tends to become. Take, for example, oats. Let's look at five ways oats can be prepared. There is a clear order of preference.

1. Oat Flour. Oat flour, being in flour form, will rapidly lose nutrients and will elevate your blood sugar quickly.

2. Instant Oatmeal. Instant oatmeal is better than oat flour. It's called "instant" oatmeal because it cooks more quickly than regular oatmeal. The problem is, it has a rather "instant" effect on blood sugar levels. Instant oatmeal makes blood sugar levels rise quickly.

3. Regular Oatmeal. Regular rolled oatmeal is similar to instant, but it's not as finely chopped. Because of this, regular oatmeal will raise blood sugar more slowly than instant oats.

4. Thick Rolled Oatmeal. Some companies, and in particular health food companies, make oatmeal that is more thickly cut than the standard

grocery store oatmeal. These raise glucose levels more slowly than regular rolled oats.

5. Steel Cut Oats. Finally, there are steel cut oats. These are the healthiest choice. Steel cut oats are thick, so they take longer to cook, and they raise blood sugar levels more slowly and gradually than rolled oats.

Whether you eat oats or some other grain, eat grains that are minimally processed and in their most natural form.

A Special Concern About Rice

Rice has long been a staple in America and many other parts of the world, especially Asia. Recently, though, rice has been the target of much criticism, and for good reason. Note this headline on the Harvard Medical School web site: "FDA warns parents about arsenic in rice cereal." Arsenic is, of course, deadly at a certain dosage. Of great concern, levels of arsenic have found their way into rice in doses that may not be deadly, but they are unacceptable and a health risk. Some companies, such as Lundberg, are aware of the problem and are working to produce rice with low levels of arsenic. Proceed carefully with rice.

What About Wheat?

Wheat is such an American staple that it's really an icon. In fact, wheat was featured on the American copper penny from 1909 to 1958, and this penny is referred to as the "wheat penny." When most people think of flour, or bread, they think of wheat.

But wheat's reputation has been pounded in recent years. One of the main voices to speak out against wheat is cardiologist William Davis, who wrote the *New York Times* best-selling book *Wheat Belly*. Dr. Davis goes so far as to name modern wheat "Frankenwheat." Modern wheat? Yes, because Dr. Davis claims, as do others, that wheat has been the victim of severe genetic modifying over the last several decades, and that this modern Frankenwheat, which has been radically changed, is responsible for a host of health problems, one of which is increased fat on our bellies.

Another problem with modern Frankenwheat is that it's much higher in gluten than wheat was before it was genetically modified. Higher gluten levels are a big problem for a portion of the population, again, creating a host of health disorders.

If you have any type of gluten sensitivity, it's best to avoid wheat completely. If you don't have gluten sensitivity, it would still be wise to proceed cautiously with wheat, checking for symptoms, noticing how you feel. Sadly, wheat as we know it is not what it used to be and should be.

Are There Safe Grains?

There are a few grains that are considered relatively safe to eat today. Perhaps the best one is quinoa, which, in reality, is actually a seed. Other grains that usually make nutritionist's lists of the safest to eat are amaranth, barley, buckwheat, bulgur, sorghum, farro, teff, oats, millet, and wild rice.

Sprouted Bread

As mentioned, it's a good idea to avoid flour as much as possible. Even whole grain flour can be a problem. But, then, what about bread? So many people like to eat bread. Are there any viable options? Thankfully, yes. Some companies make sprouted bread that is both healthy and tastes good. Among health food and nutrition circles, these breads enjoy an excellent reputation. I can vouch for them. My family enjoys sprouted bread on almost a daily basis.

There are many brands, but probably the best-known brand is Ezekiel Bread. The original Ezekiel Bread was baked to match the recipe for bread found in the Bible book of Ezekiel. (Ezekiel 4:9) There are now several flavors to choose from, including what may be our favorite, the Cinnamon Raisin English Muffins. Give sprouted bread a try. It's nutritious and delicious. You can normally find sprouted bread in health food stores, but some local supermarkets carry them too. You'll find them in the frozen foods section.

The Recommended Healthy Approach for Grains

Whether you decide to include grains in your diet is a personal choice. Grains have both an upside and a downside. Is it possible to include grains in a healthy diet? Absolutely. Grains grow in abundance, and they are here for a reason. Properly eaten, grains can be filling, nutritious, and delicious.

Still, there are a few cautions for those who eat grains. Don't let them become the staple of your diet. Vegetables should hold that position. To requote the wonderful Dr. Hyman: "As with most foods, the dose of grains is key. I recommend ½ cup to 1 cup of grains per day. If you are an athlete and are metabolically healthy (only 12 percent of us), you may be able to include more grains."

Try to select the healthiest grains. Be careful with wheat, for a host of reasons, and rice, because of the high arsenic content in modern rice. If at all possible, eat grains that have been minimally processed. And make sure to chew your grains thoroughly.

Grains are not absolutely necessary in our diets. But they can be a fine addition if you eat the right grains in the right amounts. If you do eat grains, enjoy them!

Chapter 9

Nuts and Seeds

• Nuts and seeds are generally recognized as health-promoting foods that contribute to a healthy diet. Both nuts and seeds have been called "nutritional powerhouses," due to their high nutrient density. But there are many who believe that nuts and seeds contain too much fat and are too calorically rich to be healthful. This is especially true of those who recommend extremely low-fat diets. Who is correct? Should you eat nuts and seeds as part of a healthy diet? If so, how much should you eat?

Some nutritional experts believe that nuts and seeds are too calorically dense to be regularly included in a healthy diet. For instance, popular writer Dr. John McDougall says that "these are rich foods for special occasions." Famous cardiologist Caldwell Esselstyn counsels against including nuts and seeds in the diet, citing their high fat content. Most, if not all of those who are opposed to nuts and seeds are advocates of extremely low-fat diets. (They tend to recommend a maximum dietary fat content of ten percent. At such a low rate, considering that most foods contain some fat, it's almost impossible to stay under the ten percent limit by including ANY fatty foods such as nuts and seeds, avocados, oils, etc.)

On the other hand, the vast majority of nutritionists consider nuts and seeds to be healthy additions to the diet. Some consider them optional, and some consider them essential. Joel Fuhrman, for instance, includes nuts and seeds in his catchphrase acronym "G-BOMBS." These are his daily essentials, and the acronym represents Greens, Beans, Onions, Mushrooms, Berries, and Seeds (and Nuts).

There are two low-fat nutritional experts who I'd like to take a moment to commend. They are T. Colin Campbell and Dean Ornish. Both Dr. Campbell and Dr. Ornish recommend low fat diets for overall health and heart health. Not many years ago, both were opposed to including nuts and seeds in the diet. However, they have both changed their stance. The preponderance of evidence that shows that nuts and seeds lead to better health outcomes has caused them to allow small amounts of nuts and seeds in the diet. This is nutrition at its finest. Instead of holding firmly to a position, these men have courageously adjusted their points of view to match the evidence.

Let's look at what Dr. Campbell wrote about this matter:

> But fat content aside, I am impressed with the findings now showing health benefits for most nuts. And when we judge a food by one nutrient, in this case judging nuts only because of their fat content, we may be falling into the same trap that has caused so much past misinformation.

> Being narrow minded creates problems; being broad minded solves problems. (Campbell)

Beautiful work, Dr. Campbell.

I agree with the vast majority of nutritionists who have two main beliefs regarding nuts and seeds. 1. They are nutritional powerhouses, and they should be included in most people's daily diets. 2. They are very rich—high in fat and calories—and therefore they should be eaten in moderation.

What Does the Science Show?

The Cleveland Clinic reports that the diets of 110,000 people were examined in two major studies: Nurses' Health Study and the Adventist Health Study. The results? "Those who ate 5 or more ounces of nuts per week had a substantially lower risk of heart disease and death. How much lower? People who ate more nuts lowered their risk by 35% to 50%. (Wow!)" Wow indeed! Other studies yielded similar results.

Omega-3s

A few nuts and seeds contain exceptionally high amounts of omega-3 fatty acids. Omega-3s are known to have special qualities that benefit both heart and brain health. They do this in a variety of ways, including lowering triglycerides and reducing inflammation. Omega-3s are so important to our health that even some vegan advocates recommend taking fish oil, which is outstandingly high in omega-3s, as a medicine.

While fish oil and fatty fish, such as salmon, are excellent sources of omega-3s, there are good sources among nuts and seeds. The top sources are walnuts, flax seeds, chia seeds, and basil seeds. Some find it convenient to add these nuts and seeds to their smoothies. Flax seeds are filled with omega-3s, but eating them whole does not provide omega-3 protection, as they will pass through your system whole. Flax seeds must be ground before use to access the omega-3s inside.

Brazil Nuts

Brazil nuts get a special shout out here, because they stand out among nuts in one important area. Brazil nuts are the best source of the mineral selenium. Selenium is an essential mineral that helps with hair and nail health, thyroid function, immune system protection, and reproductive health. Selenium is difficult to obtain in our diets, but just one or two Brazil nuts a day provide all the selenium we need. Some add a nut or two to their smoothies. It's important to note, though, that excessive selenium is not desirable. Chronic selenium excess can cause serious problems. If you eat Brazil nuts, it's best to limit them to one or two a day.

Should I Soak or Sprout Nuts Before Consumption?

Nuts and seeds can be difficult to digest due to their high phytic acid content. Soaking nuts and seeds breaks down and neutralizes the phytic acid, making digestion and assimilation easier and increasing nutrient absorption. Therefore, some nutritionists recommend soaking or sprouting nuts and seeds before consumption.

There are many different methods of soaking and sprouting nuts and seeds, and each nut and seed, depending on its size, will require different lengths of soaking. I recommend that you look at the various soaking and sprouting methods on the web and choose the one that you feel most comfortable using. You can also buy sprouted nuts and seeds.

Thrive Market, an online natural food store, sells an abundance of these products. As a heads up, give the brand Daily Crunch a try. The Sea Salt and Turmeric flavored almonds are amazing.

How Many Nuts and Seeds Should We Eat?

As we've discussed, nuts and seeds are a wonderful and important addition to our diets. Most nutritionists highly recommend that we include them on a daily or near-daily basis. But those same nutritionists recommend that we exercise restraint, due to the high fat and calorie content of nuts and seeds.

So how many nuts and seeds should we eat? Most nutritionists recommend about 30 grams a day, depending, of course, on your body size and your personal nutritional requirements. Thirty grams is approximately one ounce or one handful. How many nuts and seeds comprise 30 grams, or one ounce or one handful? Here's a sampling:

- 25 almonds
- 15 cashews
- 15 pecans
- 30 pistachios
- 10 walnuts
- 15 macadamias
- 3 tbsp. pumpkin seeds
- 3 tbsp. sesame seeds
- 4 tbsp. flax seeds (ground)
- 3 tbsp. chia seeds

You can overdo it when it comes to nut and seed consumption. Kathy McManus, director of the Department of Nutrition at Harvard-affiliated Brigham and Women's Hospital, reports: "If you eat more than one or two handfuls of nuts per day, you're adding extra calories—maybe too many—that can take the place of other healthy foods and add weight."

Think in terms of small portions. Have a handful of nuts or seeds for a snack. Or add a few nuts and seeds to meals throughout the day.

Raw or Roasted?

My favorite nut is cashews, and I love them roasted and with salt. That's good, but . . . will they love me back? While it's okay to have roasted nuts and seeds on occasion, raw, or uncooked, is better. Simply put, oils are not as healthy when they have been heated, and nuts and seeds have a very high oil content. That said, I eat the majority of my nuts and seeds, including cashews, raw. Taste is important, but health comes first.

Are Nut and Seed Butters Okay?

Yes, they are fine. Just make sure that the butter is pure and unhealthy substances have not been added, such as sugar, unhealthy oils, or excessive amounts of salt. Raw butters are better, but toasted or roasted are okay.

The Recommended Healthy Approach for Nuts and Seeds

Nuts and seeds are indeed little powerhouses of nutrition. They are loaded with vitamins, minerals, fiber, and healthy unsaturated fats. For the vast majority of us, they can be healthful additions to our daily diets. Studies have shown that those who eat nuts and seeds on a regular basis have better health outcomes.

But due to their calorically dense nature, it's best to eat nuts and seeds in moderation. Normally, that means a maximum of one or two ounces a day, which equals roughly one or two handfuls a day. In place of whole nuts and seeds, you can eat a couple of tablespoons of pure, high-quality nut and seed butter each day.

While it is not essential for most to do so, some soak or sprout their nuts for better digestibility.

Nuts and seeds are best eaten in their natural states, raw (not roasted) and unsalted. Nuts and seeds have a high oil content, and unheated oils are healthier than heated oils. If salt is not a problem for you, small amounts of salted nuts and seeds will provide only a small amount of salt.

Certain nuts and seeds are especially high in beneficial omega-3 fatty acids. Omega-3 fatty acids are especially healthy for the heart and brain. High omega-3 nuts and seeds include walnuts, flax seeds, chia seeds, and basil seeds. It can be very helpful to incorporate these into your daily diet.

Brazil nuts are the best dietary source of selenium. It can be helpful to have one or two Brazil nuts a day, but don't overeat these, as they are high in fat and calories, and too much selenium can be problematic.

Nuts and seeds can be eaten with any meal. They also make wonderful snacks. Just a small handful should provide enough energy and nutrients to provide power and to hold you over to your next meal.

Nuts and seeds, in moderation, are wonderful, healthful additions to the daily diet.

Chapter 10

Dairy

• Once hailed as an amazing health and bodybuilding superfood, many experts now view dairy as being unnecessary and even unfit for human consumption. Is dairy healthful, harmful, or somewhere in between?

I remember when I was a teenager circa 1974. I went with my grandmother (do I ever miss Becky!) to visit relatives in New England. We stopped at the Vermont Welcome Center as we entered Vermont from Massachusetts. (Question for Massachusetts people: Who taught you how to drive? . . . The majority of readers might be puzzled here, but drivers in the Northeastern United States are probably laughing, and applauding.) Each visitor was kindly offered a glass of fresh Vermont creamery milk. Did I ever enjoy that! It was cold and creamy and smooth as silk. Just delightful. Only about ten years earlier, when I was a small child, I remember having a strong aversion to milk, and I believe this was only strengthened when I learned where milk actually came from.

And my youthful up and down view of dairy matches how dairy has been viewed by nutritional experts during the past several decades. It's had an up and down reputation during that time period.

Just sixty years ago, milk was considered such a vital necessity that a man, called the "milkman," actually delivered bottles of fresh milk right to your door on scheduled days of the week. Now, many shun dairy milk and favor nut or grain milks instead.

But while the experts wrangle over this topic, dairy consumption has actually soared. Especially has the consumption of cheese increased, which has almost tripled in the past fifty years. Most of this is in the form of melted cheese, which finds its way in and on top of an increasing variety of foods. But the figure that I find most mind-boggling is this: dairy consumption from all forms of dairy, in the United States, is currently a whopping 655 pounds per person per year. I couldn't believe that figure, which is almost two pounds per day. But the more I researched it, the more I found other reliable sources that confirmed its accuracy.

So, what do the nutritional experts say about dairy consumption? Really, they are all over the map on this one. Vegans, of course, shun all animal products, including dairy. Notice these words of Dr. Pam Popper, who lives and teaches a vegan lifestyle. Concerning dairy products, she said:

> I think that's the most toxic of all. When I give lectures, I get asked, "If I were going to do one thing and one thing only, what would you suggest I do?" Well, one change alone won't do the trick if you're eating the standard American diet. But if you're going to make an important first step that would improve your health, get dairy out of the diet. Dairy products have no upside. (Popper)

She also says that she views the concept of humans eating dairy products as "kind of gross."

Oftentimes, the argument is made that humans are the only species that continues to consume dairy products after early childhood as well as to consume dairy from another species. That's logical . . . or is it? Notice these words by Dr. Chris Kresser, who is a leader in the field of functional medicine:

> What about the idea that humans shouldn't drink milk because no other animal drinks the milk of another animal? By this logic, we humans should also avoid cooking our food and drinking coffee and alcohol. I don't know of any other animals doing these things, but that alone is not a sufficient reason for us not to do them. We've developed both technological methods and genetic adaptations that enable us to enjoy and benefit from dairy products; other animals don't have these options, so comparing ourselves to them in this case doesn't make sense. (Kresser)

That's pretty logical too.

Is dairy necessary in the teenage or adult diet? No. Does it have any upside whatsoever? Perhaps. For instance, according to the Harvard University T.H. Chan School of Public Health: "The nutrients and types of fat in dairy are involved with bone health, cardiovascular disease, and other conditions. Calcium, vitamin D, and phosphorus are important for bone building, and the high potassium content of dairy foods can help lower blood pressure." Try making such an argument in favor of, say, a can of soda. You can't. There simply is no upside to chemical sugar water.

Dairy products make exquisite fermented foods. Dairy yogurt and kefir are enjoyed by millions. I very clearly remember a television commercial campaign in the 1970s by the Dannon yogurt company. It ran for a couple of years, and it seemed to vault yogurt from being an obscure and rather weird food right into the mainstream of the American public. I'll let Wikipedia describe the campaign:

> In the commercials, shots of elderly (Soviet) Georgian farmers were interspersed with an off-camera announcer intoning, "In Soviet Georgia, where they eat a lot of yogurt, a lot of people live past 100." Each shot had a caption at the bottom, which would tell the audience the farmer's name and his or her age, which ranged from 95 to 105. One such commercial ended with a shot of an old man eating Dannon yogurt, with a woman who was purported to be his 114-year-old mother looking at him fondly. The announcer said, "89-year old Bagrat Tabaghua... ate two cups. That pleased his mother very much." (Wikipedia)

This marketing bit of genius landed on the list of the 100 Greatest Advertising Campaigns of all time, coming in at number 89. It was brilliant, and it did wonders for Dannon's bottom line, making it very profitable. The product tasted good too; I ate them all the time.

The problem was that Dannon marketed a huge line of, maybe, 15 flavors of their cups of yogurt. One of those flavors was plain. But how much plain yogurt did they sell? The popular flavors were strawberry, blueberry, cherry, and so on. The "fruit" was on the bottom of the cup, not preblended, and it was loaded with sugar. The sugar masked the somewhat sour taste of the yogurt, but the large amount of sugar was not desirable. If you are going to eat dairy yogurt or kefir, it's better to eat it plain or with a little fruit and perhaps a dab of a natural sweetener, such as honey or maple syrup.

Dairy has a few downsides. Please note these words of wisdom from Mark Hyman: "Milk also increases insulin-like growth factor 1 (IGF-1) in humans, which is like Miracle-Gro for cancer cells. Not only does milk fail the science tests for health benefits, but also modern industrial cow dairy makes many people very sick." Sadly, cows today are not what they were many years ago. They are raised with hormones and antibiotics, and these readily flow into the milk supply. They are also under lots of stress—from the hormones, antibiotics, diet, and awful living conditions. Commercial interests focus on profit. Sadly, the health of the animal, and subsequently the health of humans, take a back seat.

Excessive dairy consumption also creates excessive mucus production. Many have noticed this when they have eaten a lot of cheese, ice cream, or other dairy product. For the next couple of days, they may have a greater flow of mucus in their throats.

The Recommended Healthy Approach for Dairy Products

Whether or not you consume dairy products is, of course, a personal choice. Some are wise to avoid dairy completely. These include those who are lactose intolerant or otherwise sensitive or allergic to dairy. (Of course, it's wise to avoid any food that you are sensitive to or that makes you feel worse when you eat it.)

As to avoiding dairy completely, as a blanket statement applied to everyone, I don't think that is necessary. As we've read, there are arguments to be made both for dairy use and against it. I believe in restricting foods only where necessary, such as in the case of foods that are clearly dangerous, such as trans fats and refined sugar. Dairy products don't have that status, and some regard dairy as a highly nutritious food.

If you do consume dairy products, I recommend getting more bang for your nutritional buck by considering using those foods that have been cultured, such as yogurt and kefir. Many find them more filling and satisfying, and they bring wonderful benefits to your microbiome.

The source of dairy products is important too. It's generally accepted that goat and sheep dairy is superior to cow's dairy. My wife and I both love goat's milk kefir. If you are going to drink cow's milk, it's best to buy milk that is organic. It's much cleaner and safer. Cow's milk can contain either A1 or A2 casein protein. Many people have a difficult time digesting A1 casein, which is the milk that is normally sold at supermarkets. Consider A2 protein milk, which is generally considered to be more healthful and compatible with our body's needs. A2 milk is clearly marked on the container. It's available at health food stores and some grocery stores. In just the last few years, more and more A2 dairy products are being produced and marketed.

Got milk? Your call. If you think it helps you and rounds out your diet, it may be fine for you, along with other dairy products, in moderate amounts.

Chapter 11

Eggs

• Eggs are another food that has had a mixed reputation for years. Some consider eggs to be a health food. Others view them as a cholesterol bomb. Are eggs, which are a popular food for breakfast, healthy to eat?

"The incredible edible egg." That was the official slogan to promote egg sales for the egg industry some years ago. Quite catchy and quite effective. This ad was created in 1976, which was an interesting time for eggs. Egg consumption had been on a downward slide for thirty years in the United States. And it was at that time when the dangers of high serum cholesterol were entering into the nation's consciousness—eggs have lots of cholesterol. Did the ad work? It seemed to, to a degree. Today, the egg industry is rather solid and steady, with the average American eating 282 eggs per year. Asian countries lead the world with an average annual consumption of 420 eggs, followed by Mexico at 397.

Of course, you want to know if eggs are healthy or not. And what about the cholesterol? Is it an issue?

Are Eggs Healthy?

The answer to this and so many questions depend upon who is asked. There is a wide range of opinions. Holding to form, I'm going to share with you what the top nutritionists believe.

I deeply respect many of the top vegan nutritionists, such as Neal Barnard, Caldwell Esselstyn, T. Colin Campbell, Michael Greger, John McDougall, Chef AJ, and the like. They all, of course, do not include eggs in their vegan diets.

Among those who are non-vegan, most of the top nutritionists seem to believe that there is more good in eggs than negatives. The one negative that is sometimes mentioned is the cholesterol. On the other hand, the positives are that eggs are high in quality protein and many other nutrients, including choline and B vitamins. They are also inexpensive sources of nutrition.

When the cholesterol scare was peaking many years ago, it was thought that eating foods with cholesterol would have the biggest impact on your own serum cholesterol levels. Subsequent research has shown that is not accurate—the fastest way to boost your cholesterol levels is by eating saturated fat. Eggs are low in saturated fat.

So, are eggs healthy? Yes, I believe they are, and they can be a fine addition to most diets.

Are Brown Eggs Better Than White Eggs?

No, they are not. Quality wise, they are equal. The color of the shell depends on the breed of chicken that produced the egg. Some breeds lay white eggs (Andalusian, Leghorn), others lay brown eggs (Sussex, Rhode Island Red). The color is just a matter of personal preference. As an interesting note, some breeds lay eggs with other colors, such as green, blue, and cream colored.

Are All Eggs the Same Quality?

No. Certain eggs are far superior to others. I live close to an area where chickens are a big industry. The way the chickens are treated is deplorable. They live in such close quarters that they are practically stacked on top of each other. They are fed foods to make them plump that are unnatural for them to eat. And they are treated with hormones to make them grow and antibiotics to protect them from their poor living conditions. Simply put, chickens that are stressed and fed hormones and antibiotics do not produce healthy eggs. And it's these eggs that are likely the ones on the shelves of your local grocery stores.

Many companies are now producing superior quality eggs from healthy chickens. These eggs will be labeled as "free range," "organic," "pastured," or "regenerative." One of our favorite egg companies, Vital Farms, produces eggs with yokes that aren't even yellow. They are vibrant orange. Why? The healthy lifestyle and diet of the chickens causes the yokes to contain more beneficial carotenoids. And those yokes are gorgeous. They are definitely more expensive than standard eggs, but they are definitely better. These eggs are available in health food stores and finer grocery stores.

The Recommended Healthy Approach for Eggs

Eggs can be a meaningful part of a healthy diet. Many find them to be delicious, and they can be served solo and cooked in a variety of ways, or they can be a part of many recipes. Eggs are low in saturated fats, are a good source of protein, and they are loaded with nutrients.

Try to buy high quality eggs that have been produced by healthy chickens. Look for eggs that are labeled as free range, organic, pastured, or regenerative. (Or a combination of those terms, such as free range AND organic.) Depending on your size and dietary needs, limit eggs to about seven a week.

Chapter 12

Meat (Beef, Poultry, Fish, Pork, etc.)

• The subject of meat probably accounts for the biggest gulf between nutritional beliefs. The range is from zero to 100, literally. Some diets allow for zero percent meat, and more than one mandate 100 percent meat. Those who are vegan and vegetarian eat no meat at all. At the other end of the spectrum, there are those on the Lion Diet and Carnivore Diet who eat only meat—though some on the Carnivore Diet allow eggs and full-fat dairy products. And, of course, most are somewhere in between those two camps. But the question is: Is meat healthy to eat, and if so, how much should you include in your diet?

"Steak and potatoes." Those were the dietary buzzwords just a few decades ago. It was thought that if everyone ate steak and potatoes regularly, even daily, they'd be big and strong and healthy their entire lives. Then, starting in the 1960s and 70s, new diets began to spring up seemingly monthly. There was the Atkins Diet, which was high in fat and protein and low in carbs. The Stillman Diet was even lower in carbs, with practically zero allowance. Then there was the Pritikin diet, which was low-fat, low-protein, and high in complex carbs. Vegetarianism gained a toehold, and veganism soon followed. Today, the number of diets is astounding. In 2023, *Parade* listed 100 different diets, but the number goes well beyond that amount. There are probably well over a thousand different diets. And each diet has its protocol for meat consumption. Let's take a look at this matter and discern the healthy way to include, or not include, meat products in your diet.

The Arguments for Meat Consumption

Those who teach that meat should be a part of our diets believe that meat provides the highest quality protein for our bodies. Meat protein, they say, is superior to plant protein, because it is more digestible and the amino acid profile is superior, therefore meat protein is better for building and repairing our muscles. But is this true?

Apparently so. There are indexes, or charts, that rate the availability to our bodies of various sources of protein. Perhaps the best scale is called the DIAAS (Digestible Indispensable Amino Acid Score). On this scale, and other scales, animal proteins consistently and significantly outscore plant proteins for digestibility and availability. Animal proteins score very high, beans score somewhat lower, and grains score even lower. So, gram for gram of protein, animal protein will be better used by our bodies to build and maintain muscle mass and strength. Note some scores from the DIAAS chart.

Food	DIAAS Score
Whole Milk	114
Eggs (Hard Boiled)	113
Beef	111
Chicken Breast	108
Tilapia	100
Canned Tuna	100
Garbanzo Beans	83
Kidney Beans	59
Peas, Cooked	58
Oats	57
Peanuts	43
Wheat	40
Almonds	40
Corn	36

Further, those who do not eat animal products and supplement properly are deficient in vitamin B12 and some other important nutrients.

The Arguments Against Meat Consumption

On the other hand, those who do not believe that humans should eat meat have, sometimes, multiple reasons for their belief. One of those is they believe that consuming meat is detrimental to the environment. Another is that they believe meat consumption is cruel. Does anyone remember the saying "animals are people too"?

This is a book about nutrition, so I'm not going to comment on any of the ethical, social, or moral issues. Each one will have to make their own decision. (And those issues can get wacky. Recently I saw an article, which I didn't bother to read, that questioned if it was ethical to eat vegetables, because vegetables have feelings too.)

But there are those, mainly among the vegan and vegetarian groups, who believe that meat is unhealthy for human consumption. Why do they believe this? There are several reasons; the most common are listed below:

- Meats tend to be high in fat and saturated fat
- Meats contain cholesterol
- Meat can cause food poisoning
- Meat can cause inflammation
- Animals are fed hormones and antibiotics that end up in our bodies
- Excessive meat could raise our IGF-1 levels, which is a cancer risk

That's quite a list, and that's not even a complete list. But are these things true? Yes, they are.

We've looked at the main pros and cons concerning meat consumption. So, what is the balanced view?

What do The Experts Say?

Let's visit a few of the top nutritional minds and see what their thoughts are concerning meat consumption, or not meat consumption. NOTE: I won't be quoting the full spectrum of views on this matter, from vegans to carnivores, because that would be a long and confusing process for you to read. Rather, I'm going to focus on the quotes that I believe come closest to the balanced and healthy view of including meat in your diet.

"Diet plays an enormous role in muscle health. Unless you get enough of the high-quality building blocks of muscle, namely protein, you can't build muscle, especially as you age. Study after study links healthy aging and the preservation of muscle mass with higher-protein diets. Meat works the best. Then chicken, then fish. Beans are last on the list. Plant proteins must be supplemented with additional amino acids or combined with animal protein to ensure they build muscle." Mark Hyman, *The Pegan Diet*

"Think of meat and animal products as condiments or, as I like to call them, 'condi-meat'—not a main course. Vegetables should take center stage, and meat should be the side dish. Servings should be 4 to 6 ounces, tops, per meal. I often make three or four vegetable side dishes." Mark Hyman *Food, What the Heck Should I Eat?*

"Nor do you have to become a vegan or vegetarian to prevent a heart attack and reduce the risk of cancer. You just have to incorporate life-enhancing, delicious, and natural plant foods and significantly cut back on animal products." Joel Fuhrman, *The End of Dieting* (Dr. Fuhrman himself adheres to a vegan diet, but he allows for small amounts of animal protein in his recommendations.)

"Plant-based diets provide inferior-quality protein and are deficient in important nutrients while being abundant in potentially harmful compounds. However, if a person eats plant-based foods in the sense of lots of plants alongside small amounts of animal foods, the deficiencies will not be there." Jayne Buxton, author of *The Great Plant-Based Con: Why eating a plants-only diet won't improve your health or save the planet*

"In the long term, both low-protein intake (or deficient amino acid profiles) from vegetarianism/veganism, and especially carbohydrate avoidance, actually cause metabolic dysfunction. Vegan and vegetarian diets typically lead to myriad micronutrient deficiencies." *Forever Fat Loss*, by Ari Whitten

"Benefits are seen in those who consume less animal protein, but not zero animal protein. China Study author, T. Colin Campbell's own work, such as this study showed that a diet of 5% animal protein turned off cancer, but 20% turned it back on in rats exposed to aflatoxin. Similarly, the work of noted longevity expert Valter Longo, advocates for eating more protein after age 65 to maintain muscle mass.

"This is not to say that a plant based diet is unhealthy or that we should all eat steak at every meal. To the contrary, research by Dr. Valter Longo, demonstrating that the amino acid profile of animal protein is inflammatory, should be taken seriously. But a vegan diet, even when done intelligently, carries with it a very real risk of nutrient deficiency, and is not the longevity 'magic bullet' many claim it to be." Dr. Aaron Gardner, BSc, MRes, PhD

"The Adventist Health Study 2, which has been following 96,000 Americans since 2002, found that the people who lived the longest were not vegans or meat-eaters. They were "pesco-vegetarians," or pescatarians, people who ate a plant-based diet including a small portion of fish, up to once daily. In other Blue Zones, fish was a common part of everyday meals, eaten on average two to three times a week." Dan Buettner, Blue Zones author and expert

"The fact is that there's nutrients we can only get from plants and nutrients we can only get from animal foods: we need both to get the full complement of nutrients that our bodies need to be healthy. Instead of fighting about whether bacon rules and vegetables suck (or vice versa), we should be celebrating the fact that the plant and animal kingdoms are both totally awesome and necessary for health!" Dr. Sarah Ballantyne

The Recommended Healthy Approach for Meat Consumption

As is often the case with nutrition, those on both sides of the issue make valid points. We want the benefits of the highest quality protein to build and maintain our muscles, but we definitely don't want to suffer from all of the negatives that were listed. The balanced approach is not only the "what," but oftentimes the answer lies in "how much."

As the quotes above show, I believe that the world's healthiest diet is much, much closer to the vegan diet. The ideal diet seems to be mostly plant-based, with just a little bit of meat and perhaps other animal products. The sweet spot may be to include animal products, by calorie count, at about five to ten or fifteen percent of your diet. That would mean you could include, perhaps once per day, a small serving of meat of about four ounces, or the size of the palm of your hand or a deck of cards. Or, you can have a serving of meat maybe three or four times a week. Some nutritionists recommend that you focus on fish, while others recommend the white meats (fish or poultry), and still others allow for and even encourage including small amounts of grassfed red meat. And as discussed in previous chapters, dairy products and eggs might be part of this equation.

This diet gives you the best of both worlds—a diet that is predominately plant based, but with enough high-quality animal protein to build and maintain good muscle mass, to avoid nutritional deficiencies, and, likely, to satisfy your appetite. That's how Blue Zones residents eat, as do many of the healthiest and long-lived people on the planet. Simply put, it works!

Below is a reprint of the objections that were listed against including meat in the diet. Notice now that the solutions are included, underlined after each objection.

- Meats tend to be high in fat and saturated fat (Eat small amounts and it won't be an issue)

- Meats contain cholesterol <u>(Eat small amounts and it won't be an issue)</u>
- Meat can cause food poisoning <u>(Cook your meat to at least the recommended temperatures, and handle and store meat properly)</u>
- Meat can cause inflammation <u>(Eat small amounts and it won't be an issue)</u>
- Animals are fed hormones and antibiotics that end up in our bodies <u>(Buy organic, grass fed, wild caught, etc.)</u>
- Excessive meat could raise our IGF-1 levels, which is a cancer risk <u>(Eat less meat when you are younger and more if you are over age 65, when IGF-1 levels drop and you need more protein)</u>

Finally, if you do eat meat, it's highly recommended that you buy the highest quality products. Select meat that is grass fed (beef), wild caught (seafood), organic, free of antibiotics and hormones.

Most people can thrive by including small amounts of meat in their diets.

SMASH

As Valter Longo and Dan Buettner point out, seafood has a special place in the diets of Blue Zone residents and other long-lived populations. Pescatarians tend to be among the healthiest people in the world. There is a wonderful acronym that is helpful in selecting fish with the highest amounts of healthy omega-3 fatty acids: SMASH. Smash stands for, Salmon, Mackerel, Anchovies, Sardines, Herring. While most wild caught seafood is considered to be health promoting, these fish in particular are known to bring exceptional amounts of cardiovascular and other benefits. Consider including them in your diet on a regular basis.

And here's my take on the two ends of the spectrum—veganism and the carnivore diet . . .

Can you be a vegan and enjoy good health? Yes, I believe that most can. It's a known fact that many vegans live long and healthy lives. But being a healthy vegan is not easy. There are lots of boxes to check to make sure that you are doing things correctly. For instance, you must take certain supplements, you must make sure that your carbs are slow carbs, you must make sure you are getting adequate protein, and you need to avoid drifting into vegan junk foods. (French fries and colas are technically vegan foods. Some even supposedly healthy vegan foods are not truly healthy.) But if you have the desire and the determination, veganism may very well be a good option for you.

Now to the carnivore diet, which is 100 percent animal products, usually meat. This is, to me, one of the biggest thumbs down I can think of. Too much protein, too much fat and cholesterol, severely lacking in certain nutrients, virtually zero carbohydrates, ZERO fiber, ZERO live food. And, to quote many a Valley Girl from the 1990s, grody to the max.

Chapter 13

Olive Oil, Other Oils

• When it comes to olive oil and other oils, there is certainly a lot of controversy and confusion among top nutritionists. The dial swings from wide left to wide right. Some recommend that we eat no oils whatsoever, including olive oil; others have very liberal views toward olive oil use. One of those is a famous cardiologist, who recommends that you "<u>drown</u> your vegetables in 100 percent olive oil." Other oils are controversial too. For instance, some consider canola oil to be a heart-healthy choice; others consider it to be toxic. Who's correct, and what's the balanced view?

"Oil bypasses the normal mechanisms of satiation. Oil is insidious; it slips under the radar, undetected by your stretch and nutrient receptors. But those additional calories from oil and other high-fat foods never go unnoticed by your ever-expanding waistline." Nutritionist and Low-Fat Vegan Proponent Chef AJ

"One of my favorite sources of heart healthy fat is olive oil, which I often call the 'secret sauce' of the Mediterranean diet. That's because olive oil contains a powerful combination of healthy monounsaturated fats and special antioxidants known as polyphenols, both of which help block the oxidation of LDL cholesterol. Olive oil also appears to help reduce inflammation, which is the real culprit behind heart disease." Cardiologist Stephen Sinatra

Let's start by considering olive oil, which is undoubtedly the king of all food oils. Note, please, the list below of prominent nutritional experts, and notice the huge variation in their views and recommendations about olive oil. (Note: The olive oil I'll be referring to in this chapter is extra virgin olive oil [EVOO], which is the highest quality olive oil.)

• **All oils, including olive oil, are not health foods. It's best to not eat any:** T. Colin Campbell, Dean Ornish, Caldwell Esselstyn, Rip Esselstyn, Joel Fuhrman, John McDougall, Michael Greger, Chef AJ

(Note: the majority of those in this group are those who recommend the low-fat vegan lifestyle.)

- **If you eat olive oil, keep it to a bare minimum**: Neal Barnard

- **Olive oil is a health food, in moderation. Eat perhaps 1-2 tablespoons a day**: Mark Hyman

- **Olive oil is healthy and is a staple in the "Blue Zones." "Drizzle" it on foods such as veggies. Perhaps eat four teaspoons a day and maybe up to a few tablespoons a day**: Dan Buettner, Blue Zones' foremost expert and author of several Blue Zones books.

- **Eat about 3 tablespoons of olive oil a day**: Valter Longo, perhaps considered the top longevity research expert in the world.

- **Olive oil is healthy. I consider it the "secret sauce" in the healthful diet of the Mediterranean region. "I drink the stuff.":** Cardiologist Stephen Sinatra.

- **"In my medical practices, I always advise my patients to get at least a liter of olive oil a week . . . It's The Ultimate Health Tool! . . . In fact, it's so good for you, I tell my patients the only purpose of food is to get olive oil into your mouth . . . Drown your vegetables in 100 percent olive oil"**: World-Renowned Cardiologist Steven Gundry.

That's a huge range, from no olive oil to at least a liter a week, which is a whopping ten tablespoons a day, and which equals over 1,200 calories daily from just olive oil alone! (Some petite people require and eat less than 1,200 *total* calories daily.) Again, all those mentioned are recognized as well-known experts in the field of health and nutrition. *And how fascinating that the last two listed, the most liberal, are prominent cardiologists.*

What Are the Potential Health Benefits of Olive Oil?

Olive oil is reported by multiple sources to provide numerous important health benefits. For instance, Fran Gage, in her book *The New*

American Olive Oil, discusses the beneficial antioxidants in olive oil. She writes: "These antioxidants circulate in the body, hooking up with free radicals, unstable compounds thought to play a role in more than 60 different health conditions including cancer and atherosclerosis, as well as aging."

A Harvard study concluded that "those with the highest intake of olive oil had a 19% lower cardiovascular disease mortality, a 19% lower risk of dying of cancer, a 29% lower risk of dying from neurodegenerative disease, and an 18% lower risk of dying from respiratory disease."

Dr. John Axe reports that studies have shown that olive oil lowers levels of LDL cholesterol and triglycerides, both known as risk factors for heart disease. At the same time, olive oil consumption has been found to raise levels of HDL cholesterol, which is the "good," or protective cholesterol. Dr. Axe also points to a study where women who consumed olive oil burned fat and lost weight.

Cardiologist Stephen Sinatra, who encourages liberal use of olive oil, calling it the "secret sauce" of the Mediterranean diet, writes that "olive oil also appears to help reduce inflammation, which is the real culprit behind heart disease."

Dan Buettner, who is the foremost Blue Zones expert, cites this glowing claim for olive oil: "Evidence shows that olive oil consumption increases good cholesterol and lowers bad cholesterol. In Ikaria (one of the five Blue Zones), for example, we found that for middle-aged people, about six tablespoons of olive oil daily seemed to cut the risk of premature mortality in half."

But Why Not Just Eat Olives?

That's a great question. And yes, olives can be considered a health food. But olives and olive oil do not have the same properties. Olives are beneficial because they contain fiber and are a whole food. On the downside, though, olives are usually cured or pickled. Those processes add a lot of sodium to the product.

The most beneficial property of olive oil is the high level of health-promoting polyphenols. When olives are cured to be sold in whole form, a large amount of the polyphenol content is lost. But those polyphenols are preserved in olive oil. Hence, olive oil has a much higher percentage of polyphenols than cured whole olives do. And that is what makes olive oil special.

The Balanced View of Olive Oil

What is the balanced view of olive oil? On this and some other controversial matters, you'll notice that I often take a stand somewhere in the middle. Why? It's not because I enjoy meekly settling for the simple compromise in situations of controversy. To the contrary, I have zero issues with sticking with the minority when that is warranted. I'll even stand on my own island if that seems right.

But in many of these food controversies, including olive oil, here's what is happening. Both sides make valid points. It's just that some have a tendency to go way overboard with their point in one direction or the other. They may have an agenda, and they develop tunnel vision. They lock in on one side of the issue, and they can't see and may not even consider the valid points that the other side makes. My goal in this book is to present the balanced, healthy view, and that often means taking the best of both sides of an argument and finding the most reasonable place in between those points of view.

And thus it is with olive oil. The side that teaches that oils are high in fat and don't provide many micronutrients for the cost of the calories makes a good point. But the side that teaches that olive oil is high in healthy fat, namely monounsaturated, and that olive oil is loaded with extremely beneficial polyphenols that promote health in a variety of ways also makes a good point. Further, there is an abundance of studies from very reputable sources, including Harvard University, which show that olive oil consumption is beneficial to health outcomes.

Therefore, I believe it's safe to say that olive oil consumption can and probably should be part of a healthy diet. I consider the sweet spot to be between one or two teaspoons and up to three or so tablespoons a day. But if you choose to do without olive oil in your diet, there is no need to fret. That's a workable option, as many have lived long and healthy lives without consuming olive oil, or even any oils, on a regular basis. Just make sure that the rest of your diet is clean and that it contains an adequate amount of healthy fats.

Am I sold on consuming a liter or more of olive oil a week? No. That seems like one of the extremes to me. Picture a huge 2-liter bottle of soda. By eating a liter of olive oil a week, that would be the equivalent of eating an excess of two of those bottles filled with olive oil every month. Wow. While polyphenols are great, the nutritional cost of eating over 1,200 calories a day in olive oil alone seems excessive. Other nutrient-rich foods would have to be left out of the diet to account for all of those calories.

What About Other Oils?

Let's take a look at the nutritional status of other seed oils. They were all the rage not many years ago. But nutritionists today are pumping the brakes, even hard. Some believe that one of the worse things you can eat is what they refer to as "industrial seed oils." Why?

Nutritionist Lindsay Christensen reports:

The conventional medical community has long promoted the idea that certain vegetable oils, also known as industrial seed oils, are "heart-healthy." The idea that these oils, which include canola, corn, peanut, safflower, sunflower, and soybean oils, are heart-healthy vegetable oils is a myth. They are only a very recent addition to the human diet, and a growing body of research indicates that they are terrible for cardiovascular health. (Christensen)

She further adds:

Vegetable oils are novel foods that have only been a significant part of the human diet for the past 150 years, a blip in our evolutionary history. A growing body of research indicates that this is no coincidence and that vegetable oil consumption may uniquely drive cardiovascular disease, rather than prevent it, through several mechanisms, including: Promoting chronic inflammation; Increasing adiposity; Increasing trans fat intake; Displacing nutrient-dense, cardioprotective foods in the diet. (Christensen)

The problem is largely how these oils are processed. Dr. Chris Kresser, who was one of the founders of the California Center for Functional Medicine, explains in an article titled "How Industrial Seed Oils are Making Us Sick." He writes:

The general process used to create industrial seed oils is anything but natural. The oils extracted from soybeans, corn, cottonseed, safflower seeds, and rapeseeds must be refined, bleached, and deodorized before they are suitable for human consumption.

- **First, seeds are gathered** from the soy, corn, cotton, safflower, and rapeseed plants.

- **Next, the seeds are heated to extremely high temperatures**; this causes the unsaturated fatty acids in the seeds to oxidize, creating byproducts that are harmful to human and animal health.

- **The seeds are then processed with a petroleum-based solvent**, such as hexane, to maximize the amount of oil extracted from them.

- **Next, industrial seed oil manufacturers use chemicals to deodorize the oils, which have a very off-putting smell once extracted.** The deodorization process produces trans fats, which are well known to be quite harmful to human health.

- **Finally, more chemicals are added** to improve the color of the industrial seed oils. (Kresser)

That does not sound very appetizing, nor healthy. How good it is to have such watchful nutritional experts pointing these things out to us, protecting our health in the process! Clearly, it would be the course of wisdom to eat only those oils that we know are health promoting. Foremost of those is probably olive oil. Other oils that are generally recognized as being health promoting are avocado, sesame, and coconut oil.

What About Cooking with Oil?

Avocado and coconut oils are both excellent cooking oils, because each has a high smoke point, which is the temperature at which an oil will begin to smoke and quickly degrade in quality. If you desire to simply coat the bottom of the cooking surface, both avocado and coconut oils are available as cooking sprays.

Olive and sesame oils have medium smoke points. You can cook with them, but only at low to moderate temperatures. Many prefer to cook in butter, which, for those who eat dairy and don't mind the saturated fat, is normally an excellent cooking option.

The Recommended Healthy Approach for Olive Oil and Other Oils

Olive oil enjoys an excellent reputation and for good reasons. Most health professionals believe that there is a definite place for olive oil in a healthy diet. Olive oil's abundance of monounsaturated fat and high polyphenol levels are reported to bring remarkable health benefits to those who consume it. Notable among these are benefits to blood lipids and the cardiovascular system.

Make sure to buy extra virgin olive oil (EVOO). All olive oils are not created equal, but there are several good brands to choose from. One very popular brand among health professionals and oil connoisseurs is California Olive Ranch.

Good olive oils will produce a characteristic bite or sting in the throat, which is caused by the polyphenols. That's a good thing.

Don't use olive oil that was harvested more than about two years earlier. And olive oil can degrade quickly after the container is opened.

Try to use containers that are small enough to allow you to finish the oil within a month or two after opening.

I recommend consuming between one or two teaspoons to as much as two or three tablespoons of olive oil a day.

Olive oil is an excellent choice when paired with vegetables, as the good fats in olive oil will help you to absorb the nutrients from the vegetables.

Other suitable oils are avocado oil, coconut oil, and sesame oil. Avocado and coconut oils are especially good for high-temperature cooking.

I recommend avoiding all "industrial seed oils." These include canola, corn, peanut, safflower, soybean, and sunflower oils. They are normally prepared at high temperatures and with toxic chemicals, which make them unfit for human consumption.

Chapter 14

Salt, Sodium

"Say 'Na' to excess sodium" – David Klein

● **Almost all nutritionists caution that too much sodium is harmful to our bodies. But how much is too much? Are certain forms of salt, such as sea salt, better than others? Do we really need to consume any salt at all? Are "salt" and "sodium" synonymous, the same thing?**

Do We Need Sodium in Our Diets?

Do we need sodium in our diets? Yes, we do. Please note this explanation from the United States Food and Drug Administration (FDA): "Sodium is an essential nutrient and is needed by the body in relatively small amounts (provided that substantial sweating does not occur) to maintain a balance of body fluids and keep muscles and nerves running smoothly." Then they mention the common problem: "However, most Americans eat too much of it—and they may not even know it." And thus it is with sodium. We need it to function optimally, but we tend to eat too much of it.

Do We Need to Add Salt to Our Foods?

Probably not. Sodium occurs naturally, in small amounts, in most foods. If we eat the amount of calories that we need, it's likely that we'll be consuming enough sodium to meet our dietary needs. However, please don't view that statement as a blanket condemnation against adding salt to our foods. It's very likely that a small amount of added salt will not be problematic for many.

Are Salt and Sodium the Same Things?

No, they are not. But they are closely related and are often used interchangeably, mistakenly, in our language. Sodium is a mineral, pure and simple. (It's chemical element symbol is "Na"—and hence, that's the origin of the corny quote at the start of this chapter.) But salt, also known as sodium chloride, is a compound consisting of 40% sodium and 60% chloride. So, salt contains a lot of sodium, but it itself is not pure sodium.

How Much Sodium Do We Need for Optimal Health?

Not nearly as much as we eat. Most adults need about 500 mg. to 700 mg. of sodium a day. The American Heart Association (AHA) recommends that we eat no more than 2,300 mg. a day, which is probably excessive. Usually, if we eat more than we need of any substance, it's not in our health's best interests. American adults consume, on average, about 3,400 mg. of sodium a day, which is far more than what our bodies need and is more than the lenient recommended limit of the American Heart Association. Our goal for optimal health should be to keep our daily sodium intake in line with our daily needs.

Where Are We Getting All This Sodium From?

The obvious answer might be the saltshaker, or even from foods we prepare at home, but that is incorrect. The majority comes from commercially prepared foods. Here are the top ten sources of sodium in the American diet, in order, according to the CDC. The first item on the list might be surprising: breads and rolls; pizza; sandwiches; cold cuts and cured meats; soups; burritos and tacos; savory snacks—including chips, popcorn, pretzels, and crackers; chicken; cheese; and eggs and omelets.

Does it Matter What Type of Salt We Eat?

The bottom line is, there is not a big difference between types of salt. Sodium chloride is sodium chloride. While it's true that natural salts, such as sea salt or Himalayan pink salts, contain minerals, the amount is very little. Regular table salt is normally iodized, meaning that the mineral iodine has been added. There's a split among nutritionists as to whether or not that's a good thing.

Most nutritionists seem to prefer sea salt or Himalayan pink salt. They believe that the small amount of minerals might be helpful and that those salts are ultimately purer.

In our home, we prefer Himalayan pink. It's gorgeous, it's pure, and it does not cost much more than regular table salt.

What Problems Arise from Eating Too Much Sodium?

Excessive sodium intake can cause serious health disorders. The most commonly known is high blood pressure, which can lead to a host of cardiac problems, including heart failure, enlarged hearts, and strokes. But too much sodium has also been linked to the following health problems: headaches, kidney disease, kidney stones, osteoporosis, and stomach cancer.

Oftentimes, the damage from excess dietary sodium takes many years to develop. Once it does, the damage is difficult to reverse. It's the course of wisdom to control sodium intake for our entire lives. If you are eating too much sodium now, this is a very good time to begin to get that under control.

Can Potassium Help?

Yes, it can. Sodium and potassium work in harmony with each other and need to be consumed in balance. Notice how this is explained by the American Heart Association:

> Potassium is a mineral that your body needs to stay healthy. Foods with potassium can help control blood pressure by blunting the effects of sodium. The more potassium you eat, the more sodium you process out of the body. It also helps relax blood vessel walls, which helps lower blood pressure. (American Heart Association)

Most people do not eat enough potassium. Here is a list of some high potassium foods: bananas, oranges, cantaloupe, watermelon, avocados, mushrooms, greens, potatoes, spinach, lentils, lima beans, raisins, tomatoes.

It should be noted that some people, including those taking certain medications, should not be eating a high potassium diet. If you have any questions about this, be certain to check with your health professional.

The Recommended Healthy Approach for Salt, Sodium

Sodium is a necessary nutrient and, in moderation, can be a delightful part of your diet. Highlighting salt's value, the word "salary" is derived from the word "salt." But too much dietary salt can cause a wide range of health problems, some of them very serious.

Most of our sodium needs can be met by the sodium that is present in natural foods. If you desire to add salt to your food, please do so judiciously—use as little as you need to enjoy your meal. If you buy prepared products, look for ones that are lower in sodium. Unless you have special needs, such as if you perspire a lot, try to keep your sodium intake to about 1,200 mg. a day or less. And again, unless you have special needs, make sure not to exceed the AHA recommended limit of 2,300 mg. a day.

Consider using natural salts, such as sea salt or Himalayan Pink.

Tip: Some find it effective to add salt to the surface of their food instead of allowing salt to be absorbed in the food items. Your taste buds have more contact with the food's surface areas. By adding salt to the surface only, you are providing your taste buds with more "bang for the buck"—more salt flavor with less total sodium.

Chapter 15

Water

"Water, water, everywhere, not a drop to drink." — Samuel Taylor Coleridge

• Is it best to drink water from the tap, from plastic bottles, or should you filter your water at home? If so, do inexpensive filters work, or do you need a more expensive one? How much water should you drink per day? Is it a good idea to drink water with meals?

Our bodies are comprised mostly of water. Naturally, if we want the fluids in our bodies to be pure, we should strive to drink pure water. But as English poet Samuel Taylor Coleridge, quoted at the outset, acknowledges, it's not always easy to find drinkable water.

A 2023 article in CNN Health by journalist Jen Christensen opened with these words: "Almost half of the tap water in the United States is contaminated with chemicals known as 'forever chemicals,' according to a study from the US Geological Survey." These forever chemicals are known as per-and polyfluorinated alkyl substances (PFAS). It's not exactly comforting to know that our water supply is tainted with "forever chemicals." But it gets worse . . .

Water from our municipal supplies is usually contaminated with many additional chemicals. These include such harmful elements as chlorine, lead, mercury, cadmium, arsenic, nitrates, nitrites, fluoride, and others, which are delivered right to our homes in our tap water.

So where can we find drinkable water?

What About Bottled Waters?

Bottled waters seem like a better idea, but the jury is still out concerning them, and the jurors don't seem to be smiling. In theory, the water is purer, as bottled water is usually spring water, distilled water, or purified water, which all should have very few contaminants. The problem with bottled water, as you probably guessed, is the container, which is more often than not made from plastic.

Let's learn more about the dangers of plastic water bottles by visiting another CNN report, this one in a 2024 article by journalist Sandee LaMotte:

> In a trailblazing study, researchers have discovered bottled water sold in stores can contain 10 to 100 times more bits of plastic than previously estimated—nanoparticles so infinitesimally tiny they cannot be seen under a microscope.
>
> At 1,000th the average width of a human hair, nanoplastics are so teeny they can migrate through the tissues of the digestive tract or lungs into the bloodstream, distributing potentially harmful synthetic chemicals throughout the body and into cells, experts say. (LaMotte)

Stunning, to say the least. And if that's not bad enough, besides these nanoplastics, there are also microplastics in plastic bottled water. So where can we get good water?

Do Water Filters Help?

Yes, they do. Even the less expensive filters, which you can buy for less than $30, do an amazing job of removing many of the contaminants in water. They are particularly effective at removing chlorine, lead, and other common seriously harmful elements. Some of the more popular low-price water filters are made by Brita, PUR, and other companies.

But there are also companies that sell higher-end filters, and these are even more efficient and can remove fluoride. Fluoride, which is good for teeth, can sadly create a host of serious problems in the body. I know that I've already shared some gruesome information about our water supply, but now that we are discussing fluoride, please read this report from the NIH (National Institutes of Health) National Library of Medicine. It opened with these words: "Recently, epidemiological studies have suggested that fluoride is a human developmental neurotoxicant that reduces measures of intelligence in children, placing it into the same category as toxic metals (lead, methylmercury, arsenic) and polychlorinated biphenyls."

Not good! So again, if you can afford a really good water filter that removes fluoride, it may be worth the investment. These filters tend to cost a few hundred dollars. Look for such names as AquaTru and Berkey, and be certain to check that they do in fact remove fluoride from your drinking water. My personal physician, who is cutting edge in these matters, recommends the AquaTru brand. We have one in our home, and we love it.

Another option is a whole house water filter.

How Much Water Should You Drink?

Lots. Most people are dehydrated. There's a simple formula that provides a general guideline as to how much water to drink: On a daily basis, you should drink half of your body weight (in pounds) in ounces of water. As an example, if you weigh 150 pounds, aim to drink 75 ounces of water a day. Of course, this is just a general guideline. You'll probably drink more in the summer months and less in the winter. And if you are involved in activities that cause you to sweat, you should drink more water accordingly.

It's a good idea to drink the majority of your water during the earlier parts of the day, as drinking too much water too late could lead to excessive nighttime urination.

Some find it convenient to buy a 32-ounce water bottle and to sip from that frequently. Doing so has two advantages. 1. It's easier to track your water when you are using a bigger container. Fill your bottle twice, and that's 64 ounces—pretty easy to keep up with. 2. If the bottle has a device that allows you to suck the water into your mouth rather than pour it, you'll probably drink more water. You may be surprised how quickly your water disappears when you do this.

Your personal water bottle should be a good quality vessel that is made of metal or a quality plastic that is BPA free. Several companies make suitable bottles.

Should You Drink Water with Meals?

It's fine to drink a little water with your meals, but only a little. Too much water with meals will dilute your digestive enzymes. Those enzymes will be less effective if they are diluted, so your digestion may be impaired. If you take digestive enzymes, then you can drink additional water.

The Recommended Healthy Approach for Water

It's very important to drink sufficient pure water. Aim to drink half your body weight (in pounds) in ounces of water daily. You can drink additional water if you desire, and especially if you are thirsty or if you are involved in activities that cause you to sweat.

You can drink a little water with meals, but too much water will dilute your digestive enzymes and render them less effective.

Tap water and water bottled in plastic are risky and even dangerous. It's preferable to get a good quality water filter and filter your tap water at home. The less expensive water filters are pretty good, but the better water filters do a superior job and can remove fluoride.

Many find it advantageous to drink from a 32-ounce water bottle. Those bottles are not very expensive. Buy a good one that's made of metal or BPA free plastic.

Water is a marvel. It's amazing that consuming a simple chemical structure, H2O, can have such a huge impact on our health. If you use a good water filter, you will find that you do indeed have sufficient water to drink, and more than just a drop!

Chapter 16

Sweeteners (Artificial and "Natural")

• Today there are sweeteners galore, including both "natural" sweeteners as well as artificial sweeteners. There's a wide range of views among nutritionists as to whether these substances are healthy. Especially is there controversy regarding artificial sweeteners. Some nutritionists view these as helpful because they are non-glycemic and might help with sugar balance and weight control. Others view them as being pure poison. Some even claim that artificial sweeteners are actually responsible for weight gain. Who is right? And what about sugar alcohols? Are they safe? What is the balanced view of using sweeteners?

Have you got a "sweet tooth"? Most people do. It starts when we are children, where our favorite foods are probably candy, cookies, cakes, pies, sodas, and ice cream. As we grow older, our sweet tooth might calm down a little, but most people still crave sweet and sugary foods, even if those foods are sweetened artificially. Sugar lights up the pleasure centers in our brains, releasing significant amounts of dopamine in the process.

There are many "natural" sweeteners, such as sucrose, honey, maple syrup, date sugar, coconut sugar, agave nectar, brown rice syrup, molasses, blackstrap molasses, sorghum syrup, monk fruit, and stevia. Then there are the artificial sweeteners, such as acesulfame potassium (Sweet One, Sunett), advantame, aspartame (NutraSweet, Equal), Neotame (Newtame), saccharin (Sweet'N Low), and sucralose (Splenda). There's a third group that essentially straddles the line between natural and artificial. They are the sugar alcohols, such as xylitol, erythritol, sorbitol, maltitol, and mannitol.

That's quite a lineup, and again, evidence that we have a collective sweet tooth.

Are Natural Sweeteners Healthy?

The short answer is that most of them can be, but only in strict moderation. Sucrose, or table sugar, however, is one of the most damaging substances ever created in a food lab. (Some consider sucrose to be more of a drug than a food.) Its addictive nature and damaging consequences have wreaked havoc on the lives of many. It's best to avoid sucrose, if at all possible. But if you have to have it, please limit sucrose to no more than a teaspoon or so a day.

Honey, pure maple syrup, date sugar, coconut sugar, agave nectar, brown rice syrup, sorghum syrup, and molasses are considered more natural than sucrose and have more redeeming qualities. For example, honey is thought to help the body in the following ways: wound healing, digestive aid, cough relief, antibacterial, antioxidant. Honey also contains some amino acids, vitamins, and minerals.

It's best, though, to learn to appreciate the natural flavors of food without adding excessive sweeteners. Even these natural sweeteners, which are almost pure sugar, will raise your glucose levels rapidly. That's why it's important to eat them only in small amounts at one time. If you do use natural sweeteners, such as honey or maple syrup, it's best to limit them to just a couple of teaspoons a day. Especially be careful with natural sugars if you have glucose or weight control issues.

Monk fruit sweetener and stevia are in a category of their own, because although they are natural sweeteners, they are not high glycemic. Neither provides calories to the body, and therefore neither will raise your blood sugar. That sounds ideal, but there are drawbacks. The most obvious drawback . . . the taste. Some don't like the taste of monk fruit or stevia. They are both sweet tasting, but both have a distinctive flavor, and usually an aftertaste, that is not present in sugar. Both stevia and monk fruit are more expensive than sugar, and stevia, in particular, can cause bloating, nausea, and gas.

Some nutritionists believe that any sweet tasting food, even if there are no carbohydrates present in that food, will trigger a release of insulin. They believe that the body is programmed, or conditioned, to anticipate that when a sweet substance is eaten that surely simple carbohydrates are part of the package and about to be assimilated. So, as a protective response, insulin will be released in the bloodstream. This, even in the absence of extra calories from the sweetener, can lead to unwanted weight gain.

Are Artificial Sweeteners Healthy?

Laboratory foods and human health are usually not compatible. And that is certainly true of artificial sweeteners, such as aspartame, (NutraSweet, Equal), saccharin (Sweet'N Low), sucralose (Splenda), and others. For instance, aspartame is classified by the World Health Organization (WHO) as "possibly carcinogenic to humans," especially with regard to risk of liver cancer. It's also been associated with increased risk of cardiovascular disease, fatty liver disease, and diabetes. According to WebMD, sucralose has been linked "to leaky gut syndrome, which means the lining of the intestines are worn down and become permeable. Symptoms are a burning sensation, painful digestion, diarrhea, gas, and bloating." It's also been referred to as a genotoxin, which is a substance that damages DNA.

Dr. Katie Page, an associate professor of medicine at the University of Southern California, makes this observation regarding artificial sweeteners:

> The more data that comes out showing these adverse health effects, the less we're going to want to encourage people to switch from added sugars to non-nutritive sweeteners . . . we really need to encourage people to eat sugar in more moderation and try to decrease sugar consumption, and the way to do that isn't to consume more non-nutritive sweeteners. (Page)

Dr. Will Bulsiewicz, who is a gut health expert and the author of the book *Fiber Fueled: The Plant-Based Gut Health Program for Losing Weight, Restoring Your Health, and Optimizing Your Microbiome*, writes the following:

> How about artificial sweeteners, ubiquitous in diet soda beverages and loads of other places? When they came to market

we thought, "Zero calories, that has to be better than sugar, right?" It's intuitive! Turns out they're actually worse because they induce changes in the microbiome that promote inflammation, insulin resistance, and liver injury. You will actually be less tolerant of sugar by using artificial sweeteners. (Bulsiewicz)

Are Sugar Alcohols Healthy?

Sugar alcohols have seen a surge in popularity in recent years. The most popular sugar alcohols today are xylitol, erythritol, sorbitol, and maltitol. Some believe that they taste more like sugar than artificial sweeteners and have less aftertaste. But are they safe to eat?

Probably not. Research is new, but it is not promising. Sugar alcohols can ferment in the gut and cause excess gas. They can also have a laxative effect. In large amounts, they can cause abdominal pain, diarrhea, and loose stools.

In a 2023 study, erythritol was linked to heart attacks and strokes. Dr. Stanley Hazen, who is a preventive cardiovascular specialist, headed this study at the famed Cleveland Clinic. He wrote: "We were looking for compounds in blood that predict risk for experiencing a future heart attack or stroke. The top candidate that kept showing up was erythritol." An interesting and mostly unknown fact is that many stevia and monk fruit products contain erythritol.

The Recommended Healthy Approach for Sweeteners

The best recommendation is to ditch the sweet tooth! I know, easier said than done. But it can be done. As you eat less sweeteners, both natural and artificial, you will begin to appreciate and enjoy the natural sweetness in foods more. You can still enjoy small amounts of the more healthful natural sweeteners, such as honey and pure maple syrup, but it's best to limit consumption to perhaps a teaspoon or two a day. And you can have small amounts of stevia and monk fruit extract if you desire. Further, you can use moderate amounts of fruits to add sweetness, such as by adding berries to a smoothie. Artificial sweeteners can be toxic and it's best to avoid those completely. Sugar alcohol may be a better option than artificial sweeteners, but they may not be safe and until proven otherwise, it may be best to avoid them too.

Chapter 17

Juices and Smoothies

• Juices were considered the ultimate health food not too long ago. They seem to have lost that polish in recent years. Smoothies are likely king today. Are juices and smoothies healthy? Should you incorporate them in your diet?

Going back a few years, juices and juice fasting were considered to be the fast track to excellent health and healing. Why did the rage begin to cool? One reason may be that while fresh vegetable juices are indeed one of the most healthful foods you can consume, people would visit the juice bars and buy, essentially, pina coladas and strawberry daquiris minus the alcohol. The vegetable juices were the true health foods, but the public sweet tooth would win out when it came time to order. And those fruit mixes were loaded with natural sugars, which would, in the long run, do more damage than good.

Smoothies are in the spotlight today. Are smoothies healthy? They can be, but the same principles apply as with juices. It's the ingredients that count, and it can be tempting to load up on carbohydrates and make the drink excessively sweet.

What is the difference between juices and smoothies? Basically, it's the pulp. The fibrous pulp is extracted from the juice and normally discarded when using a juicer, but smoothies include the pulp. Further, it's common to add other items to smoothies to make them more complete. Common ingredients added to smoothies, besides fresh produce, are protein powders, frozen fruits, nut milks, yogurt, tofu, cocoa powder, coconut water, spices, nuts and seeds (particularly flax seeds and chia seeds), and the like. If it sounds good and healthy, you can throw it in the blender. Smoothies, being so versatile and complete, are often used as convenient and healthy meals.

The Right Tools—Juicers and Blenders

It's not really practical nor cost effective to continually buy juices and smoothies at an outside establishment. It's easier and less expensive to make them yourself, and it's also safer, as you'll have full control over the ingredients and the quality of those ingredients.

Enter, the juicer and blender. If you want to make fresh juice, you'll need a juicer, and if you want to make smoothies, you'll need a blender.

There are essentially two main types of juicers, centrifugal and masticating. Centrifugal juicers are less expensive and they extract juice faster. Masticating juicers tend to cost more, they are slower, but they have a huge upside. The juice from a masticating juicer is usually of much higher quality. We have both in our home and we never use the centrifugal juicer. The quality difference is that significant. If you are going to be juicing only fruits, the difference is not great, but for juicing vegetables, and in particular leafy greens, which is possibly the most important item you could juice, the difference is dramatic. On a grade scale, I would rate the masticating juicer as an A and the centrifugal juicer as a D. (And for juicing leafy greens, the centrifugal juicer earned a big red F.) If you can afford it, then, I highly recommend a good masticating juicer. Currently, you can buy a very high-quality Omega brand masticating juicer for about $250.00 (US dollars). There are some decent cheaper brands available too.

If you want a smoothie, you'll need a blender. There is a huge price range among blenders. You can find a cheaper one for less than $30.00. The better blenders can run over $1,000.00. Again, what you can afford is at play here. And if you do plan on doing a lot of blending, making smoothies a regular feature of your diet, you'll be much happier with a good blender. Probably the premier blender brand is Vitamix. These powerful machines are used at many, and probably most, establishments that make smoothies, such as Whole Foods. A good new Vitamix will run from about $350.00 to $550.00, with some models in the range of $1,000.00. Blendtec and other companies also make popular premier blenders.

For a good blender on a budget, many prefer the Ninja models. A good Ninja costs about $100.00. I'd recommend avoiding the cheapest blenders, those that normally cost about $30.00. You'll likely be frustrated with their performance, and you may find that you are replacing those blenders, which can break under the strain of blending frozen fruits or anything that is not soft, with a new one every year or so.

Note: The Vitamix engine is so powerful that you can cook soup with the machine. I don't mean simply blend the soup; I mean <u>cook</u> it. When you run the Vitamix for a few minutes the liquid inside gets piping hot, and you can serve steamy creamed soup directly from the blender.

What If You Only Want to Buy One—a Juicer or a Blender?

Which to buy is your call, of course, but most people are happier with the purchase of a good blender. The juicer can only make juices, while some can do a few other things, such as make nut butters with a special attachment. But blenders are amazingly versatile. The choices for smoothies alone are staggering—you could have a different smoothie combination every day for scores of years. But blenders can also make so many other items. We find ways to put our Vitamix to work almost every day, and it's never let us down.

If juicing is important to you, consider buying a juicer. But if you are going to buy only one machine, and you are not sure which is more versatile, I recommend to you, without reservation, the high-speed blender.

The Recommended Healthy Approach for Juices and Smoothies

Both juices and smoothies can be wonderful additions to your diet. Juicers work by extracting the pulp and leaving just the vitamin and mineral rich liquid. Smoothies work by breaking down the fibrous pulp so that all of the liquid is released and available, mixed together with the pulp.

Both juices and smoothies can provide a huge boost to your immune system. You'll probably absorb more nutrients from a juice or smoothie than you would from eating the food whole, unless you were to chew each mouthful hundreds of times.

Be sure to juice and blend wisely. Don't include too many sweet fruits, which have quickly absorbable carbohydrates that will raise your blood sugar excessively. When you make smoothies, you can use the opportunity to blend in a good variety of healthful foods that you might not otherwise eat. Flax seeds and chia seeds work very well in smoothies, as do green drink powders and other nutrient-packed superfoods.

Also, be sure to "chew" your juices and your smoothies. You have digestive enzymes in your mouth, and by exposing the liquid to those juices, you will be giving your digestive system a helping hand.

Finally, while juices and smoothies are excellent, health-building foods, it's best to not overuse them. Make sure to eat the majority of your food from a plate or bowl, not from a glass. Normally, one glass of juice or one smoothie per day is sufficient.

Juices and smoothies, while not being a necessity for most people, can be an excellent part of a healthy diet. If you include them in your diet, may you enjoy every minute!

Chapter 18

Prebiotics and Probiotics—Gut and Microbiome Health

• Gut health was rarely written about just a few years ago, but today we hear much about it. Frequently that centers on our microbiome, which refers to the community of microorganisms, such as bacteria, fungi, and viruses, that inhabit our gut. The health of our microbiome has a huge impact on our overall health, including our digestion, immune system, and mental outlook. How can we, through our diets, keep our microbiome thriving and healthy? One powerful way is by regularly eating both prebiotics and probiotics.

What are Probiotics?

Probiotics are beneficial bacteria that exist in foods with live cultures, such as yogurt, kefir, sauerkraut, miso, kombucha, kimchi, torshi, tempeh, sour cream, aged cheeses, sourdough bread, and other similar foods. Probiotics are also available as supplements, usually in capsules. (Amazingly, just one capsule may contain over 100 billion healthy bacteria. That certainly is a huge number, but it's just a small fraction of the number contained in our guts, which, for most people, is about 100 trillion. The microbiome is just now beginning to be understood, and it is awesome.)

What are Prebiotics?

Prebiotics are foods with special plant fibers that feed the healthy bacteria in your gut. Common prebiotic fibers are inulin, fructo-oligosaccharides (FOS), and galacto-oligosaccharides (GOS). Resistant starch, though not technically a fiber, is also a prebiotic, because it behaves like a fiber. Common foods containing these fibers are garlic, chicory root, onions, Jerusalem artichokes, apples, whole oats, barley, dandelion greens, asparagus, unripe bananas (with some green still on the skin), blueberries, flax seeds, chia seeds, cooked and cooled potatoes, beans, barley, honey, and others. By including lots of natural plant foods in your diet and trying to include some of the foods listed here, you'll likely be eating sufficient prebiotics to sufficiently feed your microbiome.

Together, probiotics and prebiotics help your microbiome to thrive.

The Recommended Healthy Approach for Prebiotics and Probiotics

The recommendation is simple. Eat both prebiotics and probiotics in abundance. You can accomplish this by eating a wide variety of plant foods, including those that are known to be prebiotic foods, and by eating, preferably daily, a serving or more of probiotic (fermented) foods. You can also supplement your probiotics, if necessary, with capsules that contain a mixture of various strains of healthy bacteria.

If you are interested in learning more about how to achieve good gut health and to make your microbiome thrive, I highly recommend the book *Fiber Fueled: The Plant-Based Gut Health Program for Losing Weight, Restoring Your Health, and Optimizing Your Microbiome*, by gastroenterologist Will Bulsiewicz. He's also a top nutritionist, and he is brilliant.

NOTE: This is one of the shorter chapters in this book. But that by no means indicates that gut and microbiome health is not an important part of nutritional well-being. To the contrary, the condition of our microbiome is huge to our overall health, and pro and prebiotics are a large part of microbiome vitality. The reason this chapter is brief is that the message is simple and concise . . . The microbiome is hugely important, probiotics and prebiotics build a strong microbiome, so try to eat probiotics and prebiotics every day. Brief, simple, but very important.

Chapter 19

Vitamin and Mineral Supplements

• Are vitamin and mineral supplements really helpful? Do you need them? Which supplements should you take? What doses should you take, and how often should you take them? Are there any supplements that are best avoided?

Vitamin and mineral supplements are sold in huge quantities today. Go back about sixty years and there were very few such supplements on the market. Usually, those who used vitamin tablets took just one a day (does "One a Day" sound familiar?) of a broad-spectrum formula and that was it. One and done. Not so today. It seems that every vitamin and every variation and form of that vitamin is now available in its own bottle. You can literally fill a cabinet shelf with such supplements, and some have done exactly that. But is it necessary to do so? Is it helpful to do so? And is it even safe to do so?

There is a wide range of advice from nutritional experts regarding supplementation. Some believe that we should be able to get all the nutrients we need from our foods. Others believe that moderate supplementation is appropriate, and still others believe that substantial doses of a long list of supplements are necessary. Who is correct? Is there a balanced approach?

Why Might We Need to Supplement Our Diets with Vitamins and Minerals?

Vitamins and minerals are necessary for literally thousands of bodily functions. Deficiencies will damage our health and create all types of problems.

In an ideal world, if our health and the land and the physical and social environment were perfect, and if the foods themselves were perfect, grown on nutrient-rich, clean soil and under ideal conditions, and life was a constant stress-free joy, and we didn't get sick, grow old, and die, we'd be able to get all the nutrients we need from our foods.

Our perfect bodies would know just what to do with every nutrient we consumed. But being realistic, we certainly don't live in a world like that. The soil and foods are depleted of nutrients, our bodies are not perfect, and the stresses of this world are, at times, overwhelming. Stress depletes nutrients from our bodies.

You may find the following little quiz amazing. I sure did. I'm going to share four quotes that are all from the same source, whether that be a book or a document. Please see if you can guess the source and also the year it was published.

"Do you know that most of us today are suffering from certain dangerous diet deficiencies which cannot be remedied until the depleted soils from which our foods come are brought into proper mineral balance? The alarming fact is that foods–fruits and vegetables and grains–now being raised on millions of acres of land that no longer contain enough of certain needed minerals, are starving us–no matter how much of them we eat!"

"We know that vitamins are complex chemical substances which are indispensable to nutrition, and that each of them is important for the normal function of some special structure of the body. Disorder and disease result from any vitamin deficiency."

"Laboratory tests prove that the fruits, vegetables, grains, eggs and even the milk and meats of today are not what they were a few generations ago. No man of today can eat enough fruits and vegetables to supply his system with the mineral salts he requires for perfect health."

"Ninety-nine percent of the American people are deficient in . . . minerals, and . . . a marked deficiency in any one of the more important minerals actually results in disease."

Are you ready for the answer? Here you go. Those quotes were taken from the U.S. Senate document 264 of the 74th Congress, 2nd Session. Surprised? Maybe. But now note the date this was published . . . 1936.

Those quotes sounded so modern, but they are almost 100 years old. If this was true in 1936, how much more so nearly one hundred years later? Soils have been further depleted, and questionable farming methods have rendered the quality of our foods to be a fraction of what they should be.

Some Specific Vitamins and Minerals to Consider

It's clear that we can benefit from at least some supplementation. But what exactly should we be supplementing, and how much and how often should we be doing so? I believe you will find the answers reasonable and satisfactory.

It's essential to supplement certain micronutrients under certain conditions. For instance, the only sources of vitamin B12 are animal foods. Plants do not supply B12. If you are a vegan, you'll be severely deficient in this important vitamin if you don't supplement it. Vegans also do well to supplement with omega-3s DPA, EHA, and EPA.

There's one nutrient that we'd all likely benefit from taking. Which one? Magnesium. Why? The magnesium supply from our food sources has been severely compromised through the years. Without supplementation, it's safe to say that almost everyone is deficient in this important mineral.

Zinc is hard to get in our modern diet. What is the best source of zinc? Oysters. In the mood to down a tin of oysters? I didn't think so. Supplemental zinc will help you to stay healthy. It's difficult to get enough selenium in our diets. The best source of selenium is probably Brazil nuts. Just one or two a day will meet our selenium requirements. But many people rarely, if ever, eat Brazil nuts.

What about vitamin C? We need additional vitamin C when we are under stress or have been exposed to toxins or a virus. And then there is vitamin D. Vitamin D is actually not a vitamin at all. It's a hormone. Because it's a hormone, we can produce it within our bodies. But to do so in healthful amounts, we need copious amounts of sunlight exposure on our skin. Most don't get that in the summer and can't do that in the winter and surrounding months. Supplemental vitamin D can keep our blood levels in the proper range of this all-important hormone. And what about all of the other vitamins and minerals? Do we need to supplement them? And if so, how much and how often?

Let's get some clarity on the matter of supplementation now. This book isn't designed to dive into excessive detail, but I'll give you enough information to get you started and on your way. If you choose to go further, there are additional comprehensive sources that you can consult.

Multivitamins and minerals: We'll start with perhaps the most basic and well-known supplement . . . the multivitamin and mineral tablet (or capsule, liquid, etc.). Should you take a multivitamin? Again, the experts have varied opinions about this. Some say they are unnecessary, some say they are even dangerous, whereas others believe that it's the course of wisdom, especially with our depleted soils and food sources, to take a multivitamin every day.

One expert, longevity specialist Valter Longo, has a unique recommendation that I believe hits the balanced middle of those opinions. He recommends that we consume a diet with a high vitamin and mineral content, and that we take a supplemental multivitamin once every three days. Here's how he explains this in his book, *The Longevity Diet*: "By reducing the supplementation frequency to relatively low doses and two or three times per week, we minimize the chance of a toxic effect while still avoiding malnourishment due to a lack of a particular vitamin or mineral." Brilliant!

Even before I read this, I was practicing something similar in my routine. I use a multivitamin whose recommended daily dose is two capsules. But I didn't take two, I only took one. And I took that one not every day, but most days of the week. I recommend a similar approach for you. Make sure that you have all of the basic vitamins and minerals covered, but also make sure that you don't overdo them.

And kudos to Dr. Longo. His suggestion to take a multivitamin about half of the days of the week is nutrition at its finest . . . It's thinking outside the box, but doing so in a way that is practical, economical, and in harmony with sound nutritional principles.

A Few Multivitamin Suggestions:

Be sure to take a high-quality supplement. Try not to use just any discounted brand found on the shelf of a drugstore. All multivitamins are not created equal. If you are a man, it's normally best that your supplement does not contain iron. A multivitamin likely contains either folic acid or folate. These are actually vitamin B9. Folic acid is the synthetic form, and folate is the natural form. Try to take a multivitamin that contains the natural form, folate.

Magnesium: Magnesium is often recognized as the most common nutritional deficiency. Almost everybody could use a boost in magnesium. There are several forms of magnesium. Two very popular types are glycinate and citrate. Start out small and see how you feel. Keep in mind that taking excessive magnesium can cause loose stools. If that happens, back down your dosage. Consider a starting dose of about 200 to 300 mg. per day. Gradually work your way up to perhaps 400 to 800 mg. per day if you desire. Consider taking most of your magnesium near bedtime, as it's a known muscle and nervous system relaxant. For this reason, magnesium is found in many sleep aid formulas.

Vitamin D: As mentioned earlier, vitamin D is not a vitamin at all; it's a hormone. That's because it can be produced in the body, like the other hormones. True vitamins must be obtained through food sources.

The best way to supplement with vitamin D is to take periodic blood tests to measure vitamin D levels, and then to adjust up and down to stay in a healthful range, which is normally considered about 35 to 80 ng/ml. (Some consider 40 to 60 ng/ml to be the "sweet spot.") A supplemental dose that supplies 500 to 5,000 IU per day is common. Supplemental vitamin D is available as vitamin D-3.

If you want to increase your vitamin D naturally, you must get out in the sun and expose as much skin as possible to sunlight. Try not to wash the oils off your exposed skin for several hours after exposure, as the sun-drenched oils in your skin continue over time to produce vitamin D.

Vitamin B12: Vegans are usually very well acquainted with vitamin B12. Why? Because if they've heard it once, they've heard it a thousand times . . . we can't get vitamin B12 from plant food sources. The vegan website, www.forksoverknives.com, explains the importance of this well: "Vitamin B12 deficiency is serious and can cause anemia, nerve damage, neurocognitive changes, and, over time, paralysis—all problems that you don't need." Amen to that!

How much vitamin B12 should be supplemented? If you are not a vegan, you probably get all you need from your food, and if you take a multivitamin tablet as described above, that's even more insurance. For vegans, the usual daily dosage is in the range of 50 to 500 mcg. Importantly, as with vitamin D and other vitamins, it's a good idea to have your blood levels checked and to use that information as a guide to your dosing routine as you work with your health professional.

Omega-3s: Omega-3s are all the rage in recent years, and for good reasons. They are vital to your health.

A few nuts and seeds contain exceptionally high amounts of omega-3 fatty acids. Omega-3s are known to have special qualities that benefit both heart and brain health. They do this in a variety of ways, including lowering triglycerides and reducing inflammation. Omega-3s are so important to our health that even some vegan advocates recommend taking fish oil, which is outstandingly high in omega-3s, as a medicine.

While fish oil and fatty fish, such as salmon, are excellent sources of omega-3s, there are good sources among nuts and seeds. The top sources are walnuts, flax seeds, chia seeds, and basil seeds. Some find it convenient to add these nuts and seeds to their smoothies. Flax seeds are filled with omega-3s, but eating them whole does not provide omega-3 protection, as the seeds will pass through your system whole. Flax seeds must be ground before use to access the omega-3s inside.

Digestive Enzymes: While not technically a vitamin or mineral, digestive enzymes are commonly used and are worth a brief mention here. For those who need them, they are life savers. After years of eating foods that are difficult to digest, eating too much of those foods, eating them too frequently, and chewing them insufficiently, our digestive capabilities may diminish. Thankfully, digestive enzymes can provide what our bodies no longer can. Those who need digestive enzymes often feel a huge boost when they start taking them. Some consider their digestive enzymes to be their most important supplement. It's usually best to buy a broad-spectrum formula that assists in the digestion of each of the three macronutrients—protein, carbohydrates, and fats. I've found the Source Naturals Daily Essential Enzymes brand to be both gentle and effective. Other brands work well too.

Selenium: Selenium is known to protect the body from asthma and cancer, and it supports thyroid and reproductive health. This is the easiest mineral to "supplement" by actually eating a food. Brazil nuts are the best source of selenium, and by eating just one or two nuts a day, you should have met your selenium requirement. If you decide to supplement with selenium, it's important to keep the dose low. If you don't eat Brazil nuts, a good multivitamin-mineral tablet may provide all the selenium you need. If you do eat Brazil nuts, it's possible to ingest too much selenium. Limit them to one or two per day.

Beta Carotene: Not too many years ago, taking high doses of beta carotene was a common recommendation. Not anymore. Web MD clearly and succinctly explains the dangers of doing so, as follows:

> High doses of beta-carotene can turn skin yellow or orange. Taking high doses of beta-carotene supplements might also increase the chance of death from all causes, increase the risk of certain cancers, and possibly cause other serious side effects. Beta-carotene from food does not seem to have these effects. (Web MD)

As you read, it's best to not supplement with beta carotene. Orange foods, such as carrots, sweet potatoes, apricots, and butternut squash tend to be high in natural beta carotene.

The Recommended Healthy Approach for Vitamin and Mineral Supplements

While it's preferable to get most of your nutrients from the foods you eat, it's a fact that today's soils are depleted. Foods, even organically grown foods, do not have sufficient nutrients to supply all of our needs. Therefore, it's important to supplement wisely. Remember that the key word is "supplement"—there's no need to take massive mega-doses. You just want to make up the difference from what is missing in your food. You can consider the recommendations in the preceding pages. If you have questions, it's a good idea to speak to a health professional who is skilled in the art and science of supplementation.

Chapter 20

Fresh, Frozen, or Canned?

• Is there a place for frozen or canned foods in a healthy diet?

Fresh, frozen, or canned . . . Which is the healthiest? Often a blanket answer is given to that question. The usual answer: fresh is best, frozen next, and then, clearly the last choice, canned, which some have referred to as "dead food." However, it's not quite that straightforward, as there are situations where frozen or canned foods definitely have a place in a healthful diet.

The Recommended Healthy Approach for Fresh, Frozen, or Canned Foods

When possible, it's usually best to eat fresh foods. But that's not always possible. So here are a few tips to help you.

Produce: There's nothing like biting into a fresh piece of produce. Frozen fruit, for instance, and especially canned fruit, cannot replace the goodness, crunch, aroma, juiciness, and flavor of fresh ripe fruit. However, being realistic, sometimes you go to the grocery store and find that the tomatoes are a sickly pale pink color instead of ripe red, and they may have the consistency of cardboard. Even canned tomatoes would likely be a better choice than one of those.

And many fruits are seasonal. For instance, if you want good fresh berries, you may be confined to a small window of just a couple of months each spring or summer. If you really want those berries off season, perhaps in a smoothie, your only choice may be to buy frozen. That said, some nutritionists believe that frozen berries are as healthy as or healthier than fresh berries, even when the fresh berries are in season. Why? When berries are picked fresh, they are often picked underripe, then they are shipped to the seller, and that process may take a few days or longer. Then those berries may sit on the store shelf for several days. In the meantime, they may begin to over-ripen and even mold.

But frozen berries are usually picked ripe and then flash-frozen immediately. Those berries stay frozen until you defrost and eat them. So even though there is some loss in quality due to the berries being frozen, they are still a very high-quality product and are packed with nutrients and flavor. Personally, I prefer the taste of frozen fruits to frozen vegetables, but when fresh vegetables are not available, frozen works pretty well. As far as canned vegetables go . . . those I recommend avoiding if possible. You can see and taste that they are pretty lifeless.

Seafood: Seafood is eaten in large quantities in all three forms: fresh, frozen, and canned. In general, fresh fish is preferred to frozen fish. However, most people don't notice a huge drop-off in quality with frozen fish. Larger fish, such as tuna, salmon, and halibut are often sold frozen. And frozen fish has obvious storage and availability advantages over fresh fish. But still, for most, the goal is fresh if possible.

Tuna and salmon are two of the most popular larger fish that are sold in cans. The majority of tuna sold in supermarkets is, of course, canned. Because most people have grown up eating canned tuna, it is completely normal and natural for them. But concerning smaller fish and other seafood, such as sardines, mackerel, anchovies, and oysters, the majority of those varieties are eaten canned. They simply are not widely available fresh or frozen. If you eat seafood, it's perfectly fine to include those varieties in cans. We always have several cans of sardines, mackerel, kippers, and even oysters in our home. They are a convenient source of protein and omega-3 fats and really help out in a pinch.

As with fresh fish, it's best to buy frozen or canned fish that has been wild caught and not farm-raised.

Beans: Beans can be either cooked at home or bought in cans. Canned beans are a good buy, as they are relatively inexpensive and taste reasonably good. They are also very convenient—simply open a can and go to it. When buying canned beans, it's best to make sure that the cans are non-BPA lined. BPA lining means BPA in your food, and BPA (Bisphenol A) causes many health problems. Further, many canned beans are loaded with sodium. It's best to make sure the beans you buy have a reasonably low sodium content. Whole Foods organic line of canned beans, for instance, are reasonably priced and are low in sodium.

Of course, homemade beans are great too. You can make a big batch and refrigerate some and freeze the rest. Remember to soak the beans first, which will render them easier to cook and will lower their content of lectins, which is an unhealthful "anti-nutrient." Soak beans overnight, for up to 24 hours, for best results.

When To Eat

Meal Timing, Eating In Harmony With Your Circadian Rhythms

• **Much has been written about what we eat. And certainly, what we eat is very important. But is when we eat important? Should we eat a limited amount of meals, perhaps two or three per day, or is it okay to snack frequently, even to the point of "grazing"? Is breakfast really the most important meal of the day, or, as some suggest, should we skip breakfast and wait to eat until lunch?**

It's common knowledge that *what* we eat is important to our health and well-being. But *when* we eat is also important. Some experts believe that meal timing—when we eat and when we don't eat—is almost as important as what we eat.

How are we doing in this regard? According to the book *The P:E Diet: Leverage your biology to achieve optimal health*, by Ted Naiman and William Shewfelt, not so well. They report: "Right now, the average American is eating something with carbohydrate in it an average of EIGHT times a day, spread out over a SIXTEEN hour eating window, for a total of about 300 grams of carbs per day." That's called grazing. Dietician Julie Upton, who is the cofounder of Appetite for Health, says: "I always remind my clients that humans aren't cows. We are not meant to graze for all of our waking hours."

Cardiologist Steven Gundry, who is a huge advocate of time-restricted eating, makes this important point in his book *The Energy Paradox: What to Do When Your Get-Up-and-Go Has Got Up and Gone*: "It's not what you eat that matters most, but when and for how long you eat it that's important to how well your metabolism and energy system work."

Our Circadian Rhythms

Circadian rhythms have a profound effect on our health. What are circadian rhythms? According to the National Institutes of Health (NIH): "Circadian rhythms are the physical, mental, and behavioral changes an organism experiences over a 24-hour cycle. Light and dark have the biggest influence on circadian rhythms, but food intake, stress, physical activity, social environment, and temperature also affect them."

Circadian rhythms are abundant in the natural world around us. Most birds sing and fly during the day and go to sleep when it's dark. Those are circadian rhythms. Owls keep the opposite schedule in accordance with their own circadian rhythms. Certain flowers open during the day and close at night. Again, circadian rhythms. And our human bodies and brains are governed by circadian rhythms. We do very well to learn to live in harmony with these natural rhythms.

One of the most known circadian rhythm disturbances in humans is jet lag. Those who have flown across several times zones can tell you all about the stress of, for instance, being in a new time zone where it's the middle of the night and their bodies and brains are keyed up for full activities. Or the reverse, where they are essentially half asleep in the middle of the day. It takes several days for their bodies to adjust to the new time zones . . . which usually happens just as it's time to return home and be disoriented in the other direction.

There have been fascinating studies involving professional sport teams and circadian rhythms. Specifically, it's been found that teams based on the east coast of the United States are at a disadvantage and don't play as well when they fly to the west coast and play nighttime games. (Daytime games have little effect.) Why? Suppose the game begins at 7:30 PM and lasts until 10:30 PM. That's a pretty normal time for a sporting event for those who are based on the west coast. But for those who have just flown from the east coast, their circadian clock is viewing that as a game that started at 10:30 PM and lasts until 1:30 AM the next morning. Those players are sleepy—they literally have the sleep hormone melatonin increasing in their bodies, and their cortisol levels are very low. That does not make for optimal athletic performance. Do you think that bookies are aware of this phenomenon? Absolutely.

It's of vital importance that we eat according to natural circadian rhythms. If we don't, we will likely find ourselves in trouble. I'm speaking from experience. As a young man, I had an incident in 1980 where I took a six-hour road trip. About four hours into the trip, I decided to take a little nap. It probably would have been a good idea if I had also decided to pull off the highway and turn off my car first. Nope. I just fell asleep. Thankfully, I had little car damage and suffered no bodily harm. But it could have been a very serious situation . . . or worse. I came close to concrete pillars. But what caused that? I remember being very groggy and I remember why I was groggy. The previous evening, right before I went to sleep at about midnight, I ate a can of health-food chili. My mind and body were ready to rest, but I put a huge load on both right before I went to sleep, working against my natural circadian rhythms. When we do this, the results are never good.

Health writer and author Ari Whitten is an expert in the field of circadian rhythms and health. Note these words from his book *Eat For Energy*:

> Your circadian rhythm is the key to enjoying a healthy and vibrant life. A large and rapidly growing body of research has discovered that the circadian rhythm is a key controller of mood, motivation, body fat, metabolism, hormonal rhythms, neurotransmitter balance, cellular regeneration, sleep quality, and the health of your mitochondria—all of which have a huge impact on your energy. (Whitten)

Clearly, circadian rhythms are tied in to almost every aspect of our health and well-being. The effect is so profound, in fact, that the CDC website made this startling proclamation: "In 2007, the International Agency for Research on Cancer of the World Health Organization (WHO) announced that sufficient scientific evidence is available from animal and human studies to label shift work with circadian disruption a 'probable' carcinogen." So shift work and just being in chronic jet lag is a probable carcinogen. That's some heavy stuff!

Eating According to Your Circadian Rhythms

Now that we see how devastatingly harmful living out of harmony with your circadian rhythms can be, let's focus on what you can do to live and eat in harmony with these rhythms.

Is diet really an important factor in establishing and cooperating with your circadian rhythms? The authors of the book *Eat Like the Animals* explain it very well:

> The master body clock doesn't run as accurately as a digital wristwatch, however. It runs a little slow, so each day it needs to be reset by a reliable environmental cue. The main clock-setting cue is daylight, but the timing of eating is also important. If you subject yourself to bright light or eat when your body clock is expecting you to be asleep, you'll end up with a scrambled clock system and, ultimately, with poor health outcomes. (Raubenheimer and Simpson)

> We definitely don't want a scrambled circadian clock system. So, what can we do? Let's start by discussing breakfast.

Should You Eat Breakfast?

It's long been said that we should eat breakfast like a king, lunch like a prince, and dinner like a pauper. But it's become in vogue in recent years among some nutritional experts to recommend skipping breakfast and waiting until lunch to eat . . . or even longer. Who is correct? Should we break our fast with breakfast, or should we break our fast with lunch?

Interestingly, two of the most renowned longevity experts in the world have completely opposite views about this matter. David Sinclair, who is a professor in the department of genetics at the Paul F. Glenn Center for Biology of Aging Research at Harvard University recommends skipping breakfast. On the other hand, Valter Longo, who is a professor of gerontology and the Director of the USC Longevity Institute strongly recommends that we eat breakfast.

I could cite others who support each of these views. Who is correct? Or, perhaps the question is, who is more correct? (Arguments can be made for either point of view.) Based upon all of the reasoning and data, I'm more inclined to side with those who recommend eating a good and hardy breakfast. Let's listen to a few of their comments and you'll see why:

"While research hasn't found an exact connection, studies indicate that people who skip breakfast tend to have much higher rates of cancer, cardiovascular disease, and death. They're also more likely to have worse heart and overall health as well . . . If you're going to skip a meal, make it lunch or dinner, and definitely nix snacking before bed." Dr. Valter Longo

"It's long been known among professionals in the fitness community that eating a large breakfast is key to maintaining a lean, muscular physique. Science has confirmed that people who eat late in the day have a harder time losing weight compared to those who eat early." Mike Mutzel, *Belly Fat Effect*

"Eating breakfast regularly has been shown to help reduce the risk of developing type 2 diabetes, cardiovascular disease, and obesity. There's also evidence that eating a healthy breakfast helps with brain function, especially memory and focus." Melinda Gong, University of California Davis Health

"Eating healthy food earlier in the day is likely to fill you up and you'll be less likely to overeat in the evening. High fiber foods, healthy fats and especially lean protein, tend to suppress your appetite the most." Bodybuilder and writer Tom Venuto

"Eating breakfast provides energy to power into your day and help your body perform at its best." Cleveland Clinic Healthessentials

"Would you start a long road trip in your car with the tank on empty? Think of eating breakfast the same way. You're asking a lot of your body to get moving using only your reserves." Registered dietitian Beth Czerwony, RD, LD

We've established that eating breakfast is probably a good idea for many if not most people. What we eat for breakfast is also of keen importance. Why? If we eat too many carbohydrates, especially in the form of refined sugar and flour, we'll have an immediate rush of blood glucose that will be followed by a rush of insulin—and that will start us on an energy roller coaster for the remainder of the day. That is very stressful for the body and the mind. What's a better approach?

Jessie Inchauspé, author of *Glucose Revolution: The Life-Changing Power of Balancing Your Blood Sugar*, makes this fine recommendation: "The tradition that breakfast should be sweet is completely misguided. Build your breakfast around protein, fat, and fiber for satiety and stable energy." She adds: "An ideal breakfast for steady glucose levels contains a good amount of protein, fiber, fat, and optional starch and fruit (ideally, eaten last)." If you eat about 20-30 grams of protein at breakfast, along with a serving of healthy fat, some fiber, and perhaps a small amount of starch or fruit, your blood sugar levels will remain stable, your satiety high, and you'll feel better and eat less during the rest of the day.

All this being said, please keep in mind that it's not a good idea to eat when you aren't hungry. We have the ability to feel hunger for a reason, and that is to control when and how much we eat. So if you are not hungry in the mornings, it's okay to eat a smaller meal or to delay eating a little bit. Many wait an hour or two before they eat breakfast. Dr. Satchin Panda, who is one of the foremost leaders in the field of eating according to circadian rhythms, describes the morning as a "changing of the guard" in our bodies. Specifically, nighttime hormones, such as melatonin, rapidly decrease in the morning, and daytime hormones, such as cortisol, rapidly increase. But this takes a little time. Dr. Panda, therefore, suggests waiting an hour or two before eating breakfast to allow this change to fully develop.

How Often Should I Eat? What About Snacks and "Grazing"?

Back in the day, in the 1960s or 70s and before, it was common for people to eat "three square meals" per day. Snacking took place, a little, but it was not nearly as common as it is today. In about the 1980s, nutritional experts began to promote the idea that we all needed glucose boosts throughout the day, or we would become a nation of hypoglycemics. So, they recommended snacking between meals, making sure we eat something every two to three hours.

Somehow, two to three hours has turned, for many, into much shorter time increments. Some eat constantly all day, similar to the way cows can be seen eating grass for endless hours. Hence, the term "grazing" began to be applied to human eating habits. This way of eating has also earned a new moniker, which I find somewhat humorous: "picking and nibbling." We simply don't appear to be created to eat that way, and the health outcomes of those who do are not very good.

We want our food to provide us with nourishment and energy but not control our lives. Regularly structured meals help with this. Think in terms of fueling our vehicles. We fill them up and we go on our way until it's time to fuel them again. We don't keep hanging around gas stations, frequently stopping to top off our fuel supplies. Our bodies know how to make it from one meal to the next without frequent topping off. Jessie Inchauspé offers this simple solution: "To increase your own metabolic flexibility, eat larger, more filling meals so you don't need to snack every hour or two."

Let's take a little further look at the matter of false hypoglycemia. Please note these wise words from the book *AC: The Power of Appetite Correction* by Dr. Bert Herring. He writes:

> Hypoglycemia is the medical term for low blood sugar. Many people have a feeling of weakness and low energy several hours after eating and blame it on hypoglycemia, but this sensation, which is quite real, is almost never caused by low blood sugar. Hypoglycemia has been wrongly blamed for this feeling so often that the sensation in the absence of true hypoglycemia is called "non-hypoglycemia." Non-hypoglycemia is medical jargon meaning 'well, it's not true hypoglycemia, but it's a real sensation and we don't know exactly what causes it, so instead of calling it by a term we know to be incorrect (hypoglycemia), we'll label it "something-but-it's-not-hypoglycemia." We don't have a better

term for it, so maybe we should invent one. How about calling it the "I've taught my body to fuel up every few hours so I get jitters without a food fix blues?" Non-hypoglycemia is a wimpy weakness you can beat. Your body's better than that. Seriously, what would you do if you were in the wild for a day or two? Die after a few hours? No, your body would find its reserve and its ancient survival strength and power through the challenge. You can see for yourself by using a glucometer (the blood glucose tester that diabetics use) when the feeling occurs. If you test your blood sugar when you're feeling what you call hypoglycemia, and your blood glucose measures greater than 75 mg/dl (4.2 mmol/L), what you're feeling is non-hypoglycemia. That doesn't mean the feeling isn't real—it's just caused by something other than low glucose. Having the feeling doesn't mean it's impossible to adapt to longer intervals between eating. In fact, you can reliably overcome the feeling by insisting that your body adapt to longer intervals between eating instead of having a constant trickle of food in your gut. (Herring)

So how many times should you eat every day? A good rule of thumb is three meals or something close to that. Some prefer two meals a day, and that is probably fine. Some may eat two or three meals and a snack or even two. Especially might someone who is weak or who suffers with HPA axis disorders (adrenal output issues) need to eat smaller meals more frequently—perhaps something small every two to three hours. Experiment and see what works best for you.

On the other side of this issue is OMAD, or One Meal A Day, which has some followers. Do I recommend it? Usually not. The average person needs to eat about two thousand calories a day, and that is a lot of food to pack into one meal (and one stomach). OMAD can seem extreme and harsh, essentially undereating for 23 hours and then overeating for one hour. Three balanced meals might be the sweet spot when it comes to sensible and nutritious eating.

What About Late Evening Snacks?

Let's face it, nighttime eating is fun. But is it healthy? Generally, no. If we eat with our body's natural rhythms, we'll be eating the majority of our calories early in the day. Eating too late, even just a snack, will likely prevent us from successfully being able to practice and benefit from time-restricted eating, which we'll discuss in the next chapter. Mark Hyman, in his excellent book *Food, What the Heck Should I Eat?*, explains it this way: "Ideally you should finish dinner at six or seven p.m. and not eat again until eight or nine in the morning. That's it. It gives your body a chance to repair, heal, clean up metabolic waste in your body and brain, and more. And it stimulates weight loss."

The Recommended Healthy Approach for Meal Timing

Circadian rhythms exercise a powerful influence on our lives. According to circadian rhythm expert Dr. Sachin Panda, our brains and our bodies both have circadian rhythms. Dr. Steven Gundry reports that even our cells and microbiome have a circadian clock. Therefore, it's the course of wisdom to eat in harmony with these rhythms. Our minds and bodies are healthier and happier when we do.

This would include, if possible, eating meals on a reasonably consistent schedule. It's important to align with our clocks by eating a good breakfast, but it's usually better to do this after we have been awake for a short while, perhaps an hour or two (or less if need be), to allow our morning and nighttime hormones to have a "changing of the guard."

Grazing, or eating small amounts all day long, and eating significant food at nighttime is not in harmony with our circadian rhythms and is not healthy. It's normally best to stop eating three to four hours before you go to bed.

Eating in harmony with your circadian rhythms is an important way to fine tune your health and synch your internal clocks, enabling you to live a healthier and more robust life.

Chapter 22

Time-Restricted Eating— Intermittent Fasting

"Eating is wonderfully healthy for the body. So is fasting. Benefit from the best of both worlds on a daily basis. Eat during the day, stop eating at night, and get out of your body's way. Wonderful things will happen!" – David Klein

• **Is time-restricted eating really beneficial? How can it help you? Is an overnight fast of 12 hours sufficient, or should you aim for 14, 16, or even 18 hours or more? What about OMAD (One Meal a Day)? Is that a good idea?**

Note: The terms time-restricted eating and intermittent fasting are semi-interchangeable. I'll be using "time-restricted eating" (TRE) in this chapter, which I think is a better and more descriptive phrase.

Time-restricted eating. It's a relatively new term, but it's been practiced for millenniums. Only recently has it been tagged with a name. But is time-restricted eating a necessary or even healthful practice? If so, is there a sweet spot for the length of the restricted, or fasting, period?

What, exactly, is time-restricted eating? As the name implies, it involves eating for a specific period of time, and then refraining from eating anything caloric for another period of time. (Water, tea, and black coffee are exceptions and are usually allowed in the non-feeding window.) There is a wide variety of time-restricted eating methods being practiced. Some of the more popular are 12:12 (fasting for 12 hours and then eating for the other 12 per day), 14:10 (fasting for 14 hours and eating for the other 10), 16:8 (fasting for 16 hours and eating for the other 8), and OMAD "one meal a day" (which involves eating only one meal a day, essentially eating for perhaps 1 or 2 hours and fasting for the other 22 or 23).

Just how popular is time-restricted eating today? Dr. David Sinclair, longevity expert from Harvard University, says that "time restricted eating is the most popular diet in the world now and probably the most effective diet ever."

What does time-restricted eating do for the body? Notice these wonderfully beneficial effects, according to the NIH National Library of Medicine: "TRE reduces body weight, improves glucose tolerance, protects from hepatosteatosis (fatty liver), increases metabolic flexibility, reduces atherogenic lipids and blood pressure, and improves gut function and cardiometabolic health in preclinical studies." It also reduces the risk of diabetes, helps us on a hormonal and cellular level, improves brain function, improves sleep, elevates mood, synchs our body clocks, improves digestion, lowers inflammation, rejuvenates mitochondria, increases longevity, reduces risk of cancer, and increases overall well-being.

Which is the Preferred TRE Schedule?

Note: Before going further, please know that it is the course of wisdom, so much so that it almost doesn't even need to be said, that the fasting window should always include your night's sleep. That alone should account for perhaps six to nine hours of your fasting window. From there, it's not difficult to add in the few hours that will be needed to complete your fasting time period.

Typically, daily time-restricted eating windows run anywhere from 12 hours (12 hours fasting and 12 hours eating) all the way to OMAD, which is eating once a day for about an hour or two and fasting for the rest of the day. The most popular increments are 12:12, 14:10 (the first number is the length of the fasting window, the second the eating window), 16:8, 18:6, and OMAD. Which, though, is the preferred, or healthiest, schedule? As with everything else health and nutrition, it depends on who you ask. Some will always lean toward playing it safe, while others will tend to push the envelope.

There can be definite benefits in keeping the fast going longer. Autophagy, which is the process during fasting where the body performs cleanup and breaks down damaged and old cells and replaces them with fresh new cells, increases as the fasting window lengthens. However, the flip side is that certain risks increase as you go for longer periods without food. One of those, according to Dr. Valter Longo, who is considered by many to be the number one longevity expert in the world, is that the risk of developing gallstones increases as the daily fast goes longer. He writes: "Studies have found that people who regularly fast more than 16 or 18 hours a day have a higher risk of gallstones. They're also more likely to need surgery to remove the gallbladder. Eating for 12 hours and then fasting for 12 hours is likely safe for most people."

Many of the nutritionists whom I respect the most recommend that time-restricted eating be performed most days of the week for a minimum of twelve hours and not many more. These include Valter Longo, Joel Fuhrman, Mark Hyman, and Blue Zones expert Dan Buettner. In the Blue Zones, by the way, residents don't go out of their way to practice time-restricted eating . . . they simply just do it. It's part of the lifestyle in their communities: eat during the day and stop eating when the sun goes down. It's always better when our health routines are a way of life and not a forced activity!

There's another expert who I'd like to bring into this discussion. His name is Dr. Satchin Panda, and he is perhaps the world's foremost authority on living in harmony with circadian rhythms. He's also the author of the book *The Circadian Code: Lose Weight, Supercharge Your Energy, and Transform Your Health from Morning to Midnight.* Dr. Panda gives this advice:

> Start by establishing a 12-hour window for a week or two, and then try to decrease the time you eat by an hour a week. The reason to do this is that the optimum eating window is between 8 and 11 hours. This is because the health benefits that you get from eating within a 12-hour window double at 11 hours, and double again at 10, and so on, until you reach an 8-hour window. Eating for 8 hours or less may be feasible for some, or for many of us over a few days, but it becomes difficult for many people to sustain this over months or years. (Panda)

A fasting window of between perhaps 12 to 14 hours seems balanced and reasonable for the majority of those who are interested in the benefits of time-restricted eating. I'd recommend 12 hours as a starting point. If that works for you, and you want to try for 13 or 14 hours, that's fine too. But if 12 or 13 hours seems like your limit, that's great. You'll reap lots of benefits by doing this, and your risk will be quite low.

When Should I Begin Eating Each Day?

As we discussed in a previous chapter, it's best to begin the feeding window in the morning, perhaps within an hour or two after waking. Some try to begin their feeding window later in the day and eat deep into the evening. That's not eating in harmony with their circadian rhythms.

A Sample Day's Schedule

Let's take a sample day and see what this looks like in real life. Suppose you are following the 12:12 fasting schedule. If you begin your day with breakfast at 7:00 AM, this means that your eating window will be open for the next twelve hours, until 7:00 PM. And this is where your fasting window begins. Suppose you go to bed each night at about 10:00 PM. That's three hours fasting. And suppose you sleep for eight hours. That takes you to 6:00 AM. All you have left in the morning is one hour, which for most people is very workable.

In fact, reaching twelve hours, assuming you are in bed for at least seven to eight hours a night, comes almost automatically. The only difficult part may be to break the habit of eating a late-night snack. But notice that I wrote "habit," because a late-night snack is rarely a biological need. Once you break that habit for a few days, it becomes second nature and easy to maintain.

Who Should Not Practice Time-Restricted Eating?

As beneficial as time-restricted eating is, it's not for everyone. Here are some who would do well to avoid, or at least be cautious, with TRE:

- Those who have a history of eating disorders
- Women who are pregnant or nursing
- Those with blood sugar regulation disorders
- Those with HPA axis disorders (adrenal output issues)

If you have any concerns about time-restricted eating, you should speak with your health professional before beginning.

Do You Need to Fast Every Day?

No. You can, but it's not absolutely necessary and it's actually difficult to do. Some days it just might not work for a variety of reasons. Earthshattering? No. It's one day, so don't worry about it. Some, in fact, practice TRE maybe three or four days a week. I'd recommend more than that, especially if following the 12:12 or 13:11 patterns, because they are so easy to adhere to. But do what you comfortably and reasonably can, and you will benefit.

The Recommended Healthy Approach for Time-Restricted Eating

Time-restricted eating is all it's made out to be. It's the real deal, and it can help you in so many ways. By practicing TRE, you'll synch your all-important circadian rhythms, you'll likely lose weight, reduce your risk of heart disease and cancer, feel more energetic, strengthen your microbiome, boost your brain function and your immune system, and increase your longevity and well-being. For those who are able to do so, I highly recommend time-restricted eating.

Usually, there's no real reason to push yourself toward the longer fasting windows. Start with 12 hours, and if that becomes comfortable and you'd like to try to expand that, you may see if 13 or 14 hours works for you. By doing this, and by using your eating window to nourish your body with nutrient dense, high-quality foods, you may be amazed at how you feel.

Eating is wonderfully healthy for the body. So is fasting. Benefit from the best of both worlds on a daily basis. Eat during the day, stop eating at night, and get out of your body's way. Wonderful things will happen!

How To Eat

Chapter 23

Chewing, The Overlooked Nutritional Boost

• There's really not a lot of controversy among nutritional experts about chewing food. Most, if pressed, would say that it's beneficial to chew your food thoroughly. The problem is that this topic is almost completely ignored. Although thorough chewing provides immense health benefits, it's very rare to see a health professional recommend making this a practice. Many people, if not most, have a tendency to eat too quickly or even wolf down their foods.

Although often overlooked as a health enhancer, chewing your food thoroughly will bring you amazing benefits. Among others, here are some issues that thorough chewing helps with: digestion, weight control, resilience from disease, mental clarity, inner calm, vitality, and blood sugar balance. All that for the grand price of . . . nothing.

Chewing your food thoroughly slows down your meal, and that alone brings two main benefits: 1. It slows the release of sugar into your system. When your sugar level spikes quickly, that will be followed by a corresponding rapid insulin spike, which will in turn lower your blood sugar. That's a guarantee of one thing: that you will soon crave a quick carb fix to get your sugar back up. One rushed meal can begin an unwanted sugar high-low roller coaster throughout the entire day, or longer. Thorough chewing stretches out the meal and balances your glucose levels. 2. Your brain has built-in mechanisms to turn your hunger signal off. When you've eaten enough food, your brain sends a signal that it's time to stop eating. But that satiation signal has a time delay of several minutes. If you eat too quickly, you'll have eaten several bites (and likely hundreds of unneeded calories) before the signal has time to take effect. That leads to overeating, which, for your health, is never a good thing.

Chewing thoroughly brings other important benefits. Digesting food is quite a workload for your body. Much of our limited energy supply goes to digesting our food. True, digestion is an involuntary action, but that does not mean it's a simple or easy task for the body. Where does the digestive system begin? In the mouth. The rest of the digestive system is literally at the mercy of the mouth, because only the mouth has a voluntary role in the digestive process. Once the food gets past the mouth, it's all automatic from there. When you make the decision to chew your food thoroughly, you are aiding the digestive process in two ways:

First, and probably foremost, chewing to reduce food to small particles is absolutely vital to good digestion. Your teeth are designed to chew food; your stomach is not. If you were to forego chewing, the rest of your digestive system would have its workload multiplied exponentially. This creates a huge energy drain on your body's resources. Would you rather spend your energy in play, in getting essential work done, in spending quality time with your friends and family, or would you rather spend it digesting food that you've neglected to chew?

Second, saliva is loaded with substances that start the process of digestion right in the mouth. By breaking your food down with your teeth and saturating it with saliva, your digestive process gets a huge head start and has a much easier workload.

As an example, think, if you will, about eating a handful of cashews. (Or even try this as an experiment.) Cashews are dry, solid, and have a definite shape. But when you chew them, they quickly turn into a moist smooth paste. That's very easy work for your mouth. Picture both scenarios: either those dry, hard cashews reaching your stomach, or the smooth and liquefied cashew paste you've made with your mouth doing so. I'm sure you can see the difference from your stomach's point of view. What in the world will it do with those whole or even partially chewed cashew pieces? It doesn't have teeth and can't do the job. That food will remain largely undigested, may ferment, and will be a burden to your entire body.

Writer Aimee Gallo experimented with thorough chewing, She reports: "Most importantly: I became full on 50 – 75% less food." That, really, is a huge statement. If you think about it, who would not like to save over 50% or so on their grocery bills? And who would not want to eat less calories, be completely satisfied doing so, losing weight effortlessly in the process?

The Wisdom and Insight of Antonio and Lino Stanchich

Lino Stanchich lived a remarkable life. He died shortly before the publication of this book, at age 91. He remained active his entire life. Lino was a licensed nutritionist, educator, and author. But it's his background that set him apart and gave him such wonderful insight regarding the health benefits of thorough chewing.

Lino's father, Antonio Stanchich, was imprisoned in a WWII concentration camp in 1943. His father said that he, as was typical of all the prisoners, was "cold most of the time and hungry all the time." Prisoners were treated inhumanely, and they were provided extreme meager rations of food, causing many to starve to death. For instance, breakfast was a cup of chicory coffee and a slice of bread. Then, with those 100 calories, after freezing for the entire night, it was off to a day of hard labor.

Antonio was a resourceful man, and he tried to figure out how to make the best of, and in fact just survive, his desperate situation. He began to experiment with the way he ate his meager rations. Seemingly, the only thing he could control was his chewing technique.

Antonio started to chew each mouthful multiple times. First, he tried 50 times, then 75, then 100, 150, 200, 300 and even more. Antonio soon realized that the more he chewed his food, the better he felt. Most of his fellow prisoners scoffed at his idea, but two others were intrigued, and they joined him in his chewing sessions. All three concluded that increased chewing gave them more energy and made them feel warmer and less hungry.

And here is perhaps the most fascinating aspect of this entire ordeal. By the time the U.S. Army liberated the prisoners in 1945, only three of Antonio's crew of 32 members had survived. Which three? Antonio and the two men who joined him in his chewing experiment! Antonio credits their extensive chewing to more robust health and ultimate survival.

Shortly after he was liberated from camp, Antonio gave his son Lino the following advice: "If you are ever weak, cold, or sick, chew each mouthful 150 times or more." Lino was subsequently captured and sent to a concentration camp, and he practiced the same chewing technique. He became an expert in the matter of chewing for better health, and he shares his wealth of knowledge in his books *Power Eating Program: You Are How You Eat* and *Conscious Eating*.

In Lino's book *Conscious Eating*, he makes the following intriguing statement: "George Ohsawa, Michio Kushi, and Naboru Muramoto all write that chewing 50 times per mouthful is the basic number of chews for good digestion; 100 times or more if one has a health problem; 150 – 200 times if you have a serious sickness." The goal, of course, is to limit the amount of stress on an already stressed body by making digestion as easy as possible and to liberate maximum nutrients from the food to nourish the body.

Just one more related quote to share, this one from the *Medical Review Auschwitz*: "The veterans, more experienced prisoners, told us to take our time eating, chew our food well and for a long time. It would make us feel we had eaten more." Clearly, others in such dire circumstances, besides Antonio and Lino Stanchich, also learned the vital importance and health benefits of chewing their food thoroughly, extracting every nutrient in each bite. Thankfully, we don't have to be in such extreme circumstances to benefit from their acquired wisdom.

The Recommended Healthy and Balanced Approach for Chewing

Chew away! Make it a practice to chew each mouthful thoroughly. You'll feel so much better and be much healthier in no time if you change nothing else about your diet but this one thing.

How many times should you chew each mouthful of food? There's no specific target number, but it's safe to say that up to a certain point, the more the better.

My personal physician, wonderful Megan Anderson, of the marvelous California Center for Functional Medicine, recommends chewing each mouthful 30 to 60 times. For most people, that is a reasonable and workable goal. This amount seems to be in line with the consensus among those who recommend thorough chewing. I too recommend 30 to 60 chews per mouthful if possible. And if you feel a need to, follow the advice of Lino and Antonio Stanchich and chew even more. (Different foods require different amounts of chewing. Whatever you decide on, make sure that your solids are reduced to a paste, a liquid, or the texture of applesauce.)

But what if that seems too much for you? Perhaps you are currently eating rapidly, chewing maybe five times a bite, and you just can't see yourself reaching 30 to 60. You'll do yourself a favor by increasing to whatever amount you can. Can you double the five to ten? If so, you will reap health benefits. Can you then work up to 15 or 20? More benefits will follow.

But what if you get so hungry by mealtime that you find yourself scarfing down half your meal before you come up for air? If that's the case, Dr. Michael Lam, who recommends chewing your food at least fifty times, provides a wise solution. He suggests that, after you have eaten a portion of your meal quickly, from that point on practice thorough chewing for the remainder of the meal. (Of course, if you do feel the need to scarf down the first portion of your meal, this may be an indication that you have waited too long to eat and may have gotten overly hungry. Sometimes a little between meal or premeal snack, perhaps a handful of nuts or some raw veggies, may alleviate this problem.)

Michael Lam, by the way, is a top adrenal fatigue expert, and he cites thorough chewing as a way to improve digestion, general health, and adrenal health. Adrenal health is an important wellness issue in our stressful times. Any stress, including digestive stress, increases adrenal fatigue. By alleviating unnecessary digestive stress, you'll do yourself a favor and be rewarded with increased vitality.

Do you have to chew this many times at every meal? No, there will be exceptions. For instance, when you are dining with friends, you may not want to burden yourself with counting chews or even chewing that many times. I'd still recommend giving your food a pretty good chew even at those times, but you can do so in a way that is natural and not disruptive to the occasion.

Two more points to keep in mind. First, keep your mouthfuls of food relatively small. Chewing even fifty times probably won't get the job done if our mouths are overly stuffed. (Antonio Stanchich, when he was experimenting with thorough chewing, ate only one tablespoon of food at a time.) And finally, "chew" even your liquids, such as juices or smoothies. The mouth has essentially two jobs regarding digestion. The first is to break down food into smaller, easily swallowed particles, ideally with the goal of turning food into a paste or liquid before it's swallowed. The second is to thoroughly soak your food in saliva, which contains digestive enzymes. So even if a food is already in liquid form when you eat it, it still needs a good soaking in saliva. Hence, the very wise term: "Drink your solids and chew your liquids."

So yes, please begin to practice thorough chewing immediately. The health benefits are through the roof. It's cost-free. It will ultimately increase your joy in eating, and it will help your waistline to go down. If you do this, Antonio and Lino Stanchich would approve, and you will reap the benefits in a healthier, slimmer, and more resilient and robust you.

Chapter 24

Mindful Eating

Have you ever eaten something really good while you are watching television, and when you finish eating you realize that you paid zero attention to what you ate? It was just gone, and the experience was nil. Whenever I've done that, I feel a little sad.—David Klein, and probably most of us

• Sadly, many people in our modern world eat mindlessly. That means they are paying attention to something else while they eat, such as their phones or television screens. This leads to scarfing down food quickly, missing out on the enjoyment of the experience, and reaping less benefits from the meal. Mindful eating is a meal-enhancer.

What is mindful eating? Jeanette Wheeler Brooks of the Gaples Institute explains it wonderfully. She writes:

> Mindful eating is a simple but powerful skill that benefits both body and mind. And although we live in a fast-paced culture where distracted eating is the norm, eating mindfully is something anyone can learn with a little practice. Doing so can help you cultivate a healthier connection with your food—and more satisfaction with your meals.
>
> Mindful eating is a state of active, open awareness where you rest your attention on the full experience of eating. When we eat mindfully, we consciously observe all the sensations that arise from the aroma, taste, and texture of our food. We savor each bite without distractions. (Brooks)

What are the Benefits of Mindful Eating?

Mindful eating brings benefits to our physical, mental, and emotional health. Here are some of the benefits of mindful eating:

- We eat more slowly. This usually leads to eating less food and weight loss.

- We are motivated to prepare healthier meals.
- We enjoy the full experience of eating—the aroma, texture, and taste of the food.
- We are more cued into our hunger and satiety signals. We'll know when to stop eating.
- Our digestion gets a boost.
- We get a little break from the outside world and its stresses.
- We develop a more grateful attitude toward the provision of food. Studies show that gratitude leads to happiness.
- We develop a healthier "relationship" with food.

Tips for Mindful Eating

Here are some tips to enhance your mindful eating:

- Make your eating area comfortable. Remove distractions, such as devices.
- Pause before you begin to eat. Look at the meal, and notice the colors, textures, and shapes of the food. Consider taking a few deep breaths to help you relax.
- Chew slowly, engage your senses.
- Appreciate where the food came from, such as a garden or a local grower, and consider who prepared the meal.
- If you don't have time or the inclination to eat your entire meal mindfully, consider eating just a portion of the meal that way. Even just a few bites is helpful.

The Recommended Healthy and Balanced Approach for Mindful Eating

Mindful eating may, to some of us, initially have a "new age" sound to it, and it may therefore be a turn off. I was once of that mindset. But really, mindful eating is the way eating should be. It's our modern lifestyle that has created hurried meals, and the results have not been good. We all probably need to slow down a little, and mealtime is an excellent time to do that. The benefits to our bodies and minds are notable. If you can, begin to eat mindfully as often as possible.

Chapter 25

The Mechanics of Satiation (How to Satisfy Your Appetite Without Overeating)

● It's delightful when we eat a meal and we feel like we've eaten just the right amount of food. We are no longer hungry, and we don't feel stuffed—rather, we feel pleasingly satisfied. This is known as the Goldilocks principle: "Just Right." How can we get our satiation signals satisfied and get our meals just right, so that we don't gain weight and can lose weight if we need to?

The principles of satiation are not commonly understood, but they are actually very simple and straightforward. Let's take a look at how you can be satiated and satisfied without overeating.

What Creates Satiation?

There are two main factors that create satiation. First, you must satisfy your need for nutrients. If you are lacking in nutrients, your body and brain know it, and they will be "on the hunt" for more food. The second is that your stomach needs to stretch to a degree. These two factors work in harmony with one another and are dependent on one another to create satiety.

In other words, if you could pack all of the nutrients you need into a pill and take that pill, you would still be hungry because your stomach would be empty. On the other hand, if you ate a big meal of only popcorn, filling as it is, you would likely still be hungry for more nutrients.

Additional factors also contribute to satiation. These include taste and timing. A tasteless meal won't suffice, and neither will a meal that is over in one minute.

Our Nutrient Receptors

We have nutrient receptors in our bodies that synch with our brains and work together to let us know when we are satiated. How many different kinds of nutrient receptors are there? That's still unknown, but it's believed that we have receptors for at least each of the three macronutrients: protein, carbohydrates, and fats. If our diet is lacking in any of the three, our bodies and our brains know it. Professors David Raubenheimer and Stephen J. Simpson, authors of the book *Eat Like the Animals*, report five nutrient receptors: protein, carbs, fats, sodium, and calcium. And an argument can be made that we have more subtle receptors for many other nutrients, including vitamins.

Protein holds a special place among our nutrient receptors. Protein is satiating, it can provide fuel, and it's the only macronutrient that builds and maintains muscle. Therefore, our brains are on high alert to make sure that we consume enough protein.

I discussed this principle in the chapter "Protein," where I mentioned "protein leveraging." Here's an excerpt from that section:

> When planning your meals, it's a good idea to prioritize making sure that your protein needs have been met. That's known as protein leveraging. Those who leverage, or prioritize protein, find themselves satisfied with fewer calories in their diets and therefore are rewarded with trimmer, healthier bodies.
>
> Note: This is not to say that we should all be eating high-protein diets. We've already established that it's best to eat as much protein as our bodies need and not much more. Rather, you practice protein leveraging by simply making sure that you are meeting your protein requirement at every meal. (Klein)

Our Stretch Receptors

We also have stretch receptors in our stomachs. When our stomachs have reasonably stretched, we sense it's time to stop eating. The stretch receptors in our stomach relay that information to our brain. What's the best way to stretch our stomachs? Bulk fills our stomachs, and the bulkiest nutrient is fiber. If your stomach is filled with fiber, you'll be satiated sooner. Other foods can be filling too, of course, but fiber is the key to satiation, calorie control, and weight loss. Why? Because most of the fiber we eat is not digested—therefore, it's almost void of absorbable calories. If our stomachs are filled with high calorie foods, our stretch receptors will be activated, but at the cost of a high calorie count. So, if you increase your fiber content, you'll be satiated with less calories, and you'll love the results on your scale.

The Recommended Healthy Approach for Reaching Satiation Without Overeating

To make this easy, let's take all of the points that we've just read and put them in a numbered list.

1. Include an abundance of fiber in your diet. You can do this by eating lots of vegetables and other fibrous plant foods. I highly recommend eating non-starchy vegetables at the start of your meal, to get your stretch receptors activated as soon as possible.

2. Eat a nutrient-rich diet. And especially make sure that your protein needs are met at every meal. Along with non-starchy vegetables, I recommend eating protein at the start of the meal. By starting your meal with fibrous vegetables and protein, you'll start activating both your stretch and nutrient receptors at the beginning of your meal—and you'll quickly be well on your way to satiation.

3. Slow your meal down. Chew your food thoroughly, if you have the time, preferably 30 to 60 times per mouthful. This too will lead to increased satiation with fewer calories.

That's it. And it's really simple. But the results are astounding.

NOTE: Much to my surprise, while preparing this manuscript, I came across a diet called the "Satiating Diet." What will they think of next?

What do I think of the Satiating Diet? Actually, it's quite good. It's based on whole foods, including lean protein and fiber, and it mirrors all of the sound principles of eating that I highlight in this book. The name "Satiating Diet" fits, because it meets all of the criteria of satiation that I discuss in this chapter—it's based on lots of nutrient-rich foods and abundant fiber. Most diets are a thumbs down. This one is a thumbs up.

Part 2: Other Important Considerations

Chapter 26

The Blue Zones

• The Blue Zones are fascinating. They refer to five areas of the world where people are known to live extraordinarily long and healthy lives, featuring unusually large numbers of centenarians. By studying the Blue Zones, scientists have been able to isolate common traits, both in diet and lifestyle, that contribute to residents' vibrant health and longevity. Thankfully, we can imitate Blue Zones residents' dietary habits and reap the benefits in our own lives.

What are the Five Blue Zones?

These are the five Blue Zones:

- Okinawa, Japan
- Sardinia, Italy
- Nicoya Peninsula, Costa Rica
- Ikaria, Greece
- Loma Linda, California, United States

What are the Dietary Patterns of the Blue Zones?

While each of the individual zones has differences based on the local culture, they all have common traits. Longevity expert Valter Longo has a deep interest in the Blue Zones. In his book *The Longevity Diet,* he writes:

> Areas of the world known to have the highest prevalence of centenarians—Okinawa, Japan; Loma Linda, California; small towns in Calabria and Sardinia, Italy; and in Costa Rica and Greece—all share diets that are (1) mostly plant-based with lots of nuts and some fish; (2) low in proteins, sugars, and saturated/trans fats; and (3) high in complex carbohydrates coming from beans and other plant-based foods. Most of these centenarians ate only two or three times a day, ate light meals in

the evening, and were in many cases done eating before dark. (Longo)

That pretty well sums up the Blue Zones residents' diets. Mostly plant based. A little fish and occasional meat. Lots of beans. Enough protein, but not too much. Lots of vegetables and other complex (slow) carbohydrates. And Blue Zones residents share a Japanese saying that affects their diets in a special way . . .

Hara Hachi Bu

Blue Zones expert extraordinaire Dan Buettner explains the saying this way: "If you've ever been lucky enough to eat with an Okinawan elder, you've invariably heard them intone a Confucian-inspired phrase before beginning the meal: 'Hara hachi bu'—a reminder to stop eating when their stomachs are 80% full. Research shows it takes roughly 15 to 20 minutes for your brain to register that your stomach has reached capacity. And eating slowly, by practicing hara hachi bu, helps short-circuit this. In other words, if you stop eating when you think you're 80% full, you're likely actually 100% full (you just don't know it yet)."

Buettner mentions that the average daily caloric intake of an Okinawan is much less than that of the average American. Why? He provides a fascinating way to look at the matter. He writes: "There is a significant calorie gap between when an American says, 'I'm full' and an Okinawan says, 'I'm no longer hungry.'"

The data shows that Mr. Buettner is correct. The average American adult eats a whopping 3,600 calories per day, whereas the average Japanese adult eats 2,700. Clearly, they have different stop signals. The American stop signal is feeling 100 percent full, and the Japanese stop signal, at least for Okinawa, is feeling 80 percent full.

How many calories does the average adult need? It depends upon such matters as age, gender, size, and activity level, but 2,700 is very much in the realm of reasonableness, and 3,600 is astronomically above it.

What Other Traits Do Blue Zones' Residents Share?

Of course, this is a book about nutrition, but I'm not going to leave you hanging if you are interested in other Blue Zones' practices. Dan Buettner writes of the Power 9, or nine traits shared by residents in all of the Blue Zones:

1. **Move Naturally.** They don't pump iron or run marathons, but they stay active in their daily lives by gardening, doing house and yard work, walking, and dancing.

2. **Purpose.** They begin each morning with a sense of why they have woken up. They stay involved in purposeful activities.

3. **Downshift.** They may experience stress, but they know how and when to relax and let the stresses subside.

4. **80% Rule.** We've just discussed that one. They stop eating when they are 80 percent full.

5. **Plant Slant.** Their diets are primarily plant based. They enjoy some fish and other meats, but plants form the bulk of their diet.

6. **Wine @ 5.** They enjoy moderate amounts of alcohol, including wine, on a regular basis. (With the exception of the Adventists in Loma Linda, California.)

7. **Belong.** The vast majority of Blue Zones residents are religious.

8. **Loved Ones First.** They put their families first, including their aged parents. They commit to a life partner, and they show love and care to their children.

9. **Right Tribe.** They are either born into or form very close bonds with friends whom they are committed to for life.

What I Love About the Blue Zones

I remember the first time I heard about the Blue Zones. I was very intrigued. And since then, that intrigue has ripened to deep admiration.

The Blue Zones are not a theory and were not created in a lab. It's real life. Dan Buettner, of National Geographic, was assigned to study the longevity of residents in Okinawa, Japan, and other similar regions. He didn't have to make any suggestions or bring any elixirs. Blue Zones residents were simply living the way they and their people had been for years.

Among the most outstanding traits of Blue Zones residents are balance, modesty, and reasonableness. Nothing in their diets is "cutting edge." They don't eliminate any of the healthful food groups. They don't fear or shun any of the three macronutrients. They don't overeat. They don't practice OMAD (one meal a day). They don't graze. They do practice time-restricted eating, but in a moderate manner—usually about 12-13 hours a night. They don't eat junk food. They are not typically vegan, but their diets are primarily made up of plants—they eat meat sparingly. Their dietary habits line up perfectly with everything that I teach in this book.

Thank you for sharing Blue Zones secrets with the world, Dan Buettner.

The Recommended Healthy Approach Regarding the Blue Zones

One thing is certain, you can't argue with success. And residents of the Blue Zones are the most successful in the world at maintaining good health and living a vibrant life deep into old age, which frequently surpasses the 100-year mark.

To the extent that you can incorporate Blue Zones habits into your life, to that degree you will benefit. You can do this by eating a mostly plant-based diet, by considering eating up to a cup of beans a day, by keeping your diet low in saturated fats and free of trans fat, by nourishing your body with what you eat and avoiding sugar and all junk foods, by eating slowly and practicing hara hachi bu, which means eating only until you are 80 percent full, and by eating sparingly in the evening.

May you find delight and boost your health by living in this special, down-to-earth, time-tested way.

Chapter 27

How To Lose Weight Safely . . . And Keep it Off

"There's no such thing as a healthy overweight person, because fat on the body creates a whole constellation of pathological conditions." Dr. Joel Fuhrman, prolific author, health and longevity leader, and founder of the Nutritarian Diet

"Until you get your nutrition right, nothing is going to change." Author unknown

- **In one of the saddest situations in human history, everyone wants to be lean, look good, and feel fit. However, this seems almost impossible to accomplish, as we are getting fatter by the year. Diets and diet books abound. Countless followers adhere to their advice, yet nothing seems to work. Still, some people have managed to stay slim and fit. How do they do it? Is healthy weight loss possible? Is it sustainable? Is it bearable? And what are the keys? You'll learn how to successfully lose weight in this chapter.**

Those who have lived more than a few decades have witnessed a notable change in the body weights of perhaps themselves and definitely of those around them. If you watched a lot of television in the 1970s, 80s, and 90s, and into the early 21st century, you could not escape the endless barrage of commercials aimed at helping the masses to lose, well, mass. There were several companies vying for dominance in this dynamic business of weight loss.

This was at a time when national weight gain was just beginning. The hope was that if we followed one of these plans, we'd slim down, look great, and that would be the end of it . . . we'd remain trim and fit and beautiful for the rest of our lives. How did that work out?

It didn't. We have gained an amazing amount of weight since then, and the trend is continuing to this day. According to Joel Fuhrman, quoted at the outset of this chapter, 89 percent of the population is overweight. To make matters worse, among the 11 percent who are not overweight, most of those are alcoholics, cigarette smokers, and those with serious health problems; these ones cannot maintain a healthy weight because of those conditions. According to Dr. Fuhrman, who, by the way, I find to be an amazingly clear and brilliant educator, only 2.4 percent of American adults are in the healthy range and are, in fact, healthy. That's a national public health emergency.

One statistic that really stands out to me is the average weights of men and women today. According to the CDC, in 2018, the average adult man weighed 199.9 pounds, and the average adult woman weighed 170.8 pounds. Amazingly, the average man in the 1960s weighed 166.3 pounds. That means that the weight of the average woman today is more than the average man of just a few decades ago. Women in the 1960s (and 70s, 80s, 90s, etc.) would have been horrified to know that this trend would develop and reach this point, but it's here. The question is, can you do anything about it?

And the answer is, plenty. It's just a matter of learning what to do— learning why we gain weight and then learning how to lose weight—and then sticking with it. I'm speaking from experience. Once I learned to eat healthfully, I dropped from 225 pounds to less than 160 pounds, which was my trim young adult and even teenage weight. I can now wear the same clothing I did then. If you need to, you can achieve similar results.

Let's now look at how you can lose weight for good. We'll break this down into fourteen easy-to-follow points.

Note: Many of the fourteen points are so powerful and effective, that if you applied only one point, that would be sufficient to allow you to begin to lose weight. By incorporating most or all of the fourteen points together, you should reap amazing results.

1. You Must Have the Proper View of Food

What is food? It's a provision to do two things: 1. To nourish our bodies and provide the nutrients we need to keep us healthy—Those macronutrients, micronutrients, and phytonutrients are there for a reason. 2. Eating good food provides us with much pleasure—Our taste buds are there for a reason. Keeping those two points—nutrition and taste—in proper balance is a big key toward successful weight control.

And therein lies a big problem. Many of us, if not most of us, were taught to view food strongly through the lens of point number two. Taste, it seems, dominates most people's dietary choices. But that is a no-win situation. The Standard American Diet (SAD), also known as the Deadly American Diet (DAD), has been specifically designed to get you to eat foods that are hyperpalatable and unhealthy. Large food corporations pay scientists millions of dollars a year to develop foods that are extremely tasty and addictive. Yes, literally addictive. These foods provide very few nutrients and yet are loaded with the taste enhancers refined sugar, flour, oils, chemicals, and salt.

The health destroying view that many approach life with is to eat the best tasting foods, giving little consideration to the nutritional quality of those foods. But what is the healthy view? It's to select foods that are nutrient dense and otherwise nutritionally sound, and then eat those foods with enjoyment.

You may feel that this is an impossible task, perhaps because your taste buds have been used to eating those hyperpalatable foods for many years. But please be assured, in just days you'll begin to adjust to healthy foods, and in just a few weeks you'll be finding delight in eating a healthy diet. You'll also feel much, much better, as your health improves and you watch the pounds begin to drop off. It's a win-win situation, and I hope you go for it!

2. Eat According to Your True Hunger

Eating is enjoyable and it should be a highlight of each day. However, eating should not be viewed as a standalone recreational activity.

For instance, eating out of boredom is never a good idea. When we are bored, we can walk, read, ride a bicycle, visit a friend, create artwork, play music, watch an uplifting video, whatever. None of those activities put calories in our stomachs that end up as excessive body fat. But eating out of boredom is fraught with danger. For instance, if we are not hungry when we start eating out of boredom, how do we know when to stop? There is no stop signal because there was really never a green light in the first place. Eating when we are not hungry, whether out of boredom or not, destroys the feedback loops that are designed to keep us healthy and trim.

It's best to eat only when you are hungry and then to stop eating when you are no longer hungry. Doing so works in harmony with our built-in feedback systems that are designed to keep us at our ideal weight. The more you practice eating only when you are hungry, the more in tune you will become with your natural hunger and satiation signals.

NOTE: Eating only when you are hungry does not mean that you can't eat on a regular schedule. In fact, those who eat regular meals at regular times tend to be healthier than those who do not. You make this work by adjusting how much you eat at each meal according to your hunger. For instance, if you are only slightly hungry at mealtime, that might indicate that you ate a little too much at your previous meal. So for this meal, you can compensate and match your hunger by eating a little less than normal. By making such adjustments when necessary, you'll find that eating on a schedule works well. In no time, you'll learn to become skilled at knowing how much to eat at any given meal.

3. Eat Nutrient-Dense Foods

Foods that are high in nutrients do wonderful things for us. They provide the vitamins, minerals, and phytonutrients we need to stay healthy. We have built-in nutrient receptors in our digestive systems and our brains. That means that our brains are constantly monitoring to make sure we have eaten the proper amount of nutrients according to our needs. When we have eaten the nutrients we need, our nutrient receptors are satisfied and are "quiet." But when we have not eaten the nutrients that we need, our nutrient receptors are chattering, or even screaming, for more nutrients and more food.

So, you can see the wisdom in making sure that your food choices are nutrient dense. If we eat food that is not nutrient dense, we are literally always hungry, and we'll be craving and seeking more food in order to get more nutrients. Likely we'll give in to that, but the chances are good that we'll choose more food that is devoid of nutrients. Hence, the cycle continues, and the weight keeps packing on, and the health issues, such as diabetes, mount. But if we eat nutrient dense foods, the stop eating signal becomes clearer and more defined. No need to eat any more; no more overpowering cravings. Hence, weight maintenance and even weight loss will follow!

What are nutrient dense foods? Basically, they are foods that are in their natural, unprocessed states. Vegetables, fruits, legumes, nuts and seeds, unprocessed grains, and perhaps healthy fish, meats, eggs, and dairy provide the nutrients you need to satisfy your nutrient receptors and control your weight.

Much has been written about this subject, but I'll wrap this point up with a quote from a colleague for whom I have great admiration. He is a nutritional engineer, and his name is Marty Kendall. I mention him a few times in this book. In his book *Big Fat Keto Lies*, he writes: "The best-kept weight-loss secret is simple: if you want to lose fat, you must control your appetite by finding a way to get more nutrients per calorie from the food you consume!" Amen to that!

4. Eat Whole Foods

Eating whole foods leads to weight loss. The more fractioned, or refined our foods are, the more we tend to overeat them. Drs. Goldhamer and Lisle make this point in their book *The Pleasure Trap: Mastering the Hidden Force that Undermines Health & Happiness*: "The average overweight person, eating to full satiation on whole natural foods, will lose between 5 to 10 pounds per month. And then they will keep it off, as long as they consume a diet of whole, natural foods."

Ari Whitten, in his book *Forever Fat Loss*, adds this: "Higher intake of whole foods and higher protein intake are both—in and of themselves—known to cause a spontaneous reduction in total calorie intake of hundreds of calories per day. People lose weight not due to anything related to insulin or carbohydrates, but simply due to higher protein intake and higher whole food intake driving down their total daily calorie intake."

Those who eat whole foods lose weight by eating less calories. Compare, for example, carrots and carrot juice. Three large carrots provide 89 calories. A small eight-ounce glass of carrot juice provides 94 calories. Those three carrots will be more satiating than the cup of juice, providing less calories in the process. The fiber in the carrots makes them more filling than the juice.

And it is definitely the course of wisdom to avoid junk foods—which are not whole, are not natural, and are usually packed with excess calories—as often as possible.

5. Follow this Blue Zones' Rule: Eat Until You are 80 Percent Full

The Blue Zones are known as the healthiest regions in the world. Blue Zones residents live extraordinarily long lives, and they remain in good health well into old age. They also remain trim their entire lives. One Blue Zones region is Okinawa, Japan. And there is a Japanese saying that actually defines eating not just in Okinawa, but in the four other Blue Zones regions as well. It's called hara hachi bu, which, when translated means: "Eat until you're 80% full."

Why is this important? Slightly undereating, and I stress the word "slightly," is one of the best health secrets in the world. Eating the exact amount of calories that you need is not a bad idea either, if that were even possible. It's not, because you would be a little off the mark in one direction or the other, either over or under. To play it safe, aiming to eat until you are 80% full will help ensure that you don't exceed your needs and do not add unwanted weight.

Blue Zones expert Dan Buettner eloquently explains it this way: "If you've ever been lucky enough to eat with an Okinawan elder, you've invariably heard them intone a Confucian-inspired phrase before beginning the meal: 'Hara hachi bu'—a reminder to stop eating when their stomachs are 80% full. Research shows it takes roughly 15 to 20 minutes for your brain to register that your stomach has reached capacity. And eating slowly, by practicing hara hachi bu, helps short-circuit this. In other words, if you stop eating when you think you're 80% full, you're likely actually 100% full (you just don't know it yet)."

Buettner mentions that the average daily caloric intake of an Okinawan is much less than that of the average American. Why? He provides a fascinating way to look at the matter. He writes: "There is a significant calorie gap between when an American says, 'I'm full' and an Okinawan says, 'I'm no longer hungry.'"

Perhaps even better than aiming to stop eating when you are 80% full is to stop eating when you are no longer hungry. Your body is equipped with at least three different kinds of satiation feedback loops: nutrient receptors, stretch receptors, and YOWEL receptors. (YOWEL stands for "You're Over Weight, Eat Less." YOWEL receptors instruct us to eat less food if we are overweight. They work only when the individual is otherwise eating healthfully. Those who regularly indulge in junk foods and who eat when they are not hungry will have lost touch with the subtle signals from their YOWEL receptors.) When these receptors are all working in harmony with each other and are in rhythm, you'll know when you are hungry and when you are no longer hungry. Learn to recognize and follow these signals. Or stop eating when you are 80% full. By doing this, while eating a nutrient-rich diet, you'll guard yourself against overconsuming calories and will successfully avoid unwanted weight gain.

6. Apply the Principles of Meal Satiation

When you understand how satiation works, and you eat in harmony with that knowledge, you are well on your way to being satisfied at each meal with less food. This will, of course, help you to lose weight. This material was covered in detail in the chapter "The Mechanics of Satiation (How to Satisfy Your Appetite Without Overeating)." If you'd like more information, please refer to that chapter. But here it is in a nutshell.

Our bodies have been marvelously designed in so many ways. One of those ways is that we have appetite feedback loops. We have both nutrient receptors and stretch receptors in our bodies. These provide information to our brains to let us know when it's time to stop eating.

When both your nutrient and your stretch receptors have been satisfied, you get the signal that you've eaten a sufficient amount at any given meal. Your nutrient receptors can sense the kinds of foods you've eaten. Are they nutrient rich? What is the macronutrient balance? Do you need more protein, more fats, more carbs, more minerals, and so on. Your nutrient receptors are especially on the alert to make sure that you've had enough protein at each meal.

When your stomach has stretched to a certain degree during a meal, that information is also provided to the brain and is your other cue that you are satiated and can stop eating. The best nutrient to stretch your stomach at a minimal caloric cost is fiber. Lots of fiber will help you to feel more full, therefore more satiated, and it will lead to weight loss.

In summary, when your diet is nutrient rich, and it includes a lot of fiber, both your nutrient and stretch receptors will be satisfied, and you'll stop eating before you've overconsumed calories. So it's a good idea to make sure that, early in your meal, you put this information into practice. How can you do so?

Notice the brief summary below that explains how to satisfy your receptors early in each meal.

1. Include an abundance of fiber in your diet. You do this by eating lots of vegetables. I highly recommend eating non-starchy vegetables at the start of your meal, to get your stretch receptors activated as soon as possible.

2. Eat a nutrient-rich diet. And especially make sure that your protein needs are met at every meal. Along with non-starchy vegetables, I recommend eating protein at the start of the meal. By starting your meal with fibrous vegetables and protein, you'll be well on your way to satiation.

3. Slow your meal down. Chew your food thoroughly, preferably 30 to 60 times per mouthful if you have the time. This too will lead to increased satiation with fewer calories.

That's it. And it's really simple. But the results are amazing. You may find that applying this point alone is enough to begin a significant pattern of weight loss.

7. Chew Well and Eat Slowly

One of my favorite chapters in this book is titled "Chewing, The Overlooked Nutritional Boost." Thorough chewing, which will automatically slow down your meal, brings huge and perhaps unexpected benefits. When you chew your food thoroughly, you digest your food better and absorb more nutrients. That will satisfy your nutrient receptors and cause your cravings for additional food to diminish. Chewing thoroughly also lengthens your meal. This too will lead to greater eating satisfaction: you'll feel as though you have eaten more and will be satisfied with less food. Writer Aimee Gallo, who experimented with thorough chewing, observed this very thing. She writes: "Most importantly: I became full on 50-75% less food."

Top nutritional experts recommend that you chew each mouthful 30 to 60 times. Solid foods should be reduced to a paste, a liquid, or to the consistency of applesauce before you swallow them. Thorough chewing can not only help you to lose weight, but it will boost your overall health and well-being. Give it a try, and if you haven't done so already, I suggest you read the chapter "Chewing, The Overlooked Nutritional Boost."

8. Eat in Harmony with Your Circadian Rhythms, Including Practicing Time-Restricted Eating

Eating in harmony with our circadian rhythms brings many health benefits. One of those benefits is better body weight control. (Actually, the argument can be made that when *any* area of our health is improved, whether that be our microbiome, our sleep, our exercise habits, and even our mental and psychological condition, weight control becomes easier and improves too. As my lovely wife says, "It's all interrelated.") Let's revisit a quote from the chapter about circadian rhythms by Ari Whitten in his book *Eat For Energy*:

> Your circadian rhythm is the key to enjoying a healthy and vibrant life. A large and rapidly growing body of research has

discovered that the circadian rhythm is a key controller of mood, motivation, body fat, metabolism, hormonal rhythms, neurotransmitter balance, cellular regeneration, sleep quality, and the health of your mitochondria—all of which have a huge impact on your energy. (Whitten)

Yes, eating in harmony with your circadian rhythms will have a definite effect on your body weight. What steps can you take? This is discussed in more detail in the chapter "Meal Timing—Eating in Harmony With Your Circadian Rhythms," which I encourage you to read if you have not yet done so. But let's go over the main points:

1. Eat breakfast every day, usually within an hour or two of rising. Make sure that your breakfast has a significant amount of protein, usually 20 to 30 grams. Include some fiber and healthy fats. The protein, fiber, and fat will keep your blood sugar levels steady throughout the morning and rest of the day. You can include some carbohydrates too, but make sure they are slow carbs from natural sources. Avoid sugary foods.

Mike Mutzel, in his book *Belly Fat Effect*, makes the following point: "It's long been known among professionals in the fitness community that eating a large breakfast is key to maintaining a lean, muscular physique. Science has confirmed that people who eat late in the day have a harder time losing weight compared to those who eat early." Follow his advice, and make sure to get your day off to a healthy and nutritious start.

2. Practice time-restricted eating. It's recommended that, for most days of the week, you have an eating window of between 10 to 12 hours and a fasting window of between 12 to 14 hours. This is called "time-restricted eating," or "intermittent fasting," and it's a great way to line up with your circadian rhythms and to lose excess body weight. This is how residents of the Blue Zones eat, and it's very effective in promoting health and weight loss.

Note: Time-restricted eating may not be advisable for everyone. The following should not practice time-restricted eating, or at least should be cautious with it:

• Those who have a history of eating disorders

- Women who are pregnant or nursing

- Those with blood sugar regulation disorders

- Those with HPA axis disorders (adrenal output issues)

If you have any questions, check with your health professional before practicing TRE.

3. Eat most of your food early in the day. Avoid eating too much at night. This is called "front-loading" calories. We tend to be more active during the day, and that is the ideal time to supply our bodies with energy and nutrients. At nighttime, and especially when we are asleep, we need to use our energy to rest and to repair, not to digest food.

Practice these three simple steps involving eating with your circadian rhythms, and you will find the weight dropping off and your overall health improving.

9. To Access Your Fat Storage, Let Your Other Energy Tanks Run Low

I absolutely love the wonderful images in this section, which were created by Marty Kendall, who is an engineer living in Australia. Marty has devoted his life's work to applying the principles of engineering to nutrition. He absolutely nails this illustration. And I'm thankful to him that he has kindly granted me permission to reprint these images in this book.

Fuel Tanks Full

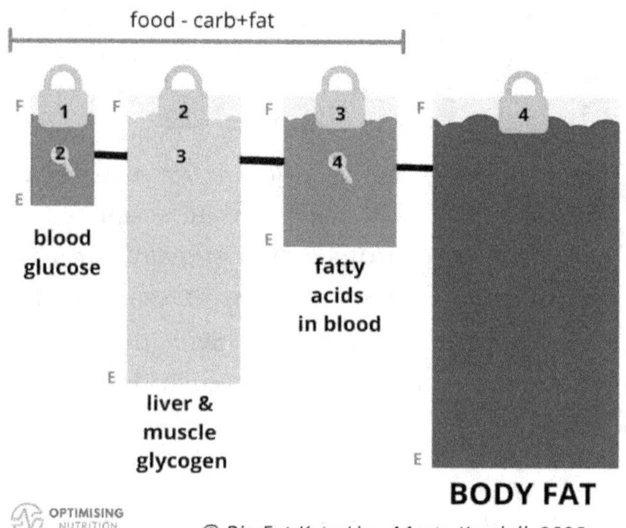

Fuel Tanks Empty

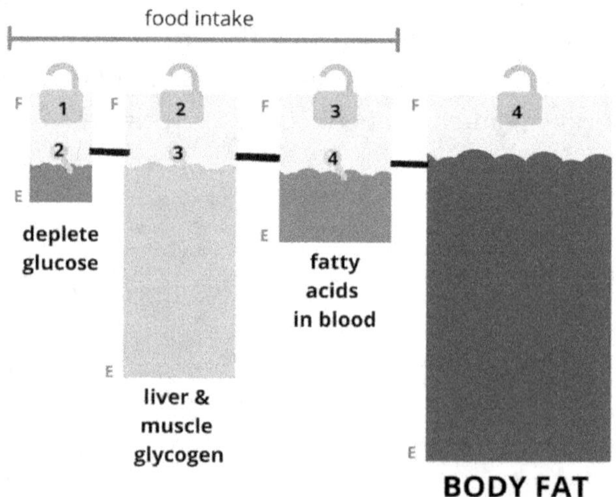

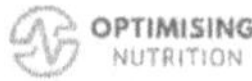

Note please that in each image, which represents our body's energy system, there are four fuel tanks. They are as follows:

1. Our blood glucose, or the sugar that is circulating in our bloodstreams.

2. The energy stored as glycogen in our liver and muscles.

3. The fatty acids in our blood.

4. Our store of body fat.

Of course, this chapter is centered on losing weight, so our focus is: How can you tap into the fourth tank, body fat, and drain some of the energy in that tank so that you lose unwanted weight? Let's dive in and show you how to begin to reduce your storage of fat.

In the illustration "Fuel Tanks Full," notice that all of the tanks are full, and the body fat content is high, filled to the brim. This means that your body is flooded with too much food energy: You have an abundance of glucose in your blood, glycogen in your liver and muscles, and fatty acids in your blood.

As long as your first three fuel tanks are all full, you'll never be able to lose weight, not even an ounce. Here's why . . . Your body has a priority list for burning fuel. And it goes exactly in the order of the tanks that Marty has created, left to right. Your body's first priority is to burn blood glucose. If there is sufficient glucose to burn, that's the easiest fuel for you to burn and it's priority number one.

When extra glucose has been depleted, your body next accesses the fuel stored as glycogen in the liver and muscles. The glycogen was formed and stored in the liver and muscles from previous meals when you ate an excess of energy. It's there as a backup, to be liberated as soon as excess glucose is burned. Your stores of both glucose and glycogen are limited, and when they are depleted, your body looks to the third option for fueling you and keeping you going. What's that? You guessed it, tank number three, fatty acids in the blood. That too is a fairly limited source. And when the first three tanks have been reasonably depleted, that's when your body looks to source number four, your storage of body fat.

So, as you can see, there is only one way to access your body fat, and that is to allow your other stores of energy to run low enough so that your body turns to tank number four for fuel. When you access tank number four, your store of body fat, you'll begin to burn that fat.

Keep in mind that none of the tanks will run completely empty. For instance, you really wouldn't feel very good if your blood sugar emptied out to zero!!! It doesn't need to do that for you to access your body fat stores. But when your blood sugar drops to levels close to your normal fasting range, that's when the next tank is accessed. The same holds true of your glycogen and fatty acids. They don't drop to zero before you move to the next tank. When the level reaches a reasonable threshold, your body knows what to do and when to do it. It moves on to the next tank.

Now let's look at the other chart, "Fuel Tanks Empty." Notice that the first three tanks are low. That means that your body fat can be accessed and burned. This chart indicates that process has indeed been happening—notice that the body fat tank has begun to go down. This is the key to losing weight. Your body needs to run through the progression of reasonably emptying the first three tanks. How does it do that?

Simply put, you can't overeat, and you can't eat too often. If you do, the first three tanks will always be full. So there need to be time periods when your energy intake is less than your energy output. What are the best ways to do this? Thankfully, we've already covered them in this book. To recap:

1. Control meal size by eating until you are 80 percent full or you are no longer hungry.

2. Be judicious with snacking, if you snack at all.

3. Avoid all addictive junk foods, especially those loaded with the sugar/fat high calorie combo.

4. Eat high nutrient, whole foods.

5. Practice time-restricted eating.

That's it in a nutshell. Again, thanks to Marty Kendall for such superb work on these charts. Marty is brilliant, and not only did he do a marvelous job on his book, *Big Fat Keto Lies*, but he also publishes a wealth of wonderful web articles further explaining the matter of weight control. You can access this site at https://optimisingnutrition.com/. I highly recommend his work to you.

10. Keep Your Macronutrients in Balance, Prioritize Protein

To lose weight effectively, you must eat a reasonable balance of macronutrients.

You want to prioritize protein in your diet. That does not mean that you should be on a high protein diet. It does mean that you should give high priority to eating the amount of protein that your body needs every day and at each meal. Why is this important?

If, for instance, you start your day without adequate protein, your energy will likely begin to wane soon after. Especially do you want to avoid a high carbohydrate breakfast, which will start you on a day of roller coaster blood sugar levels and excessive food cravings.

At each meal, make sure that you eat enough protein, that you eat non-starchy carbohydrates, that you eat a serving or so of a healthful fat, and then round out each meal with as many carbohydrates as you need to feel reasonably strong and energized until you eat again.

Marty Kendall, who I've mentioned in this book a few times, has observed that his clients who successfully lose weight have done so by prioritizing protein. They eat all of the protein that they need, and they add to that only the amounts of carbs and fats that they require to stay healthy and function properly. He explains it this way: "When we eat, we need to get sufficient protein and nutrients. You can think of carbs and fat as fuel, and we don't need as much of it if we are already carrying a lot of unwanted body fat on our body and a build-up of glucose in our liver and blood." Marty, by the way, recommends that if there is a need to cut back on food energy from carbs and fat, that it be done so gradually, or, as he calls it, 'dialing it back.'

By centering your meals on protein, non-starchy vegetables, and healthy fats, you'll be putting yourself in a position to have a good macronutrient balance and to lose weight. You can still have starchy vegetables, fruits, and whole grains, but add those judiciously, being careful not to overeat those foods, as they can raise your energy levels rapidly.

11. Stabilize Your Blood Glucose

As blood glucose levels stabilize, weight begins to drop. This material is covered more fully in the chapter "Stabilize Your Blood Glucose," so this will be a brief summary of that information. I'll reprint the key points from that chapter, which are provided courtesy of the California Center for Functional Medicine (September 2022 Newsletter)

• "Have a high-protein breakfast. Aim to consume 20-30 grams of protein to improve blood sugar control throughout the rest of the day. Then, aim for at least 4-5 oz of protein per meal for the rest of the day.

• "Always eat carbohydrates with protein, fat, and/or fiber. This helps slow the absorption of carbohydrates into the bloodstream, preventing a large spike in glucose after eating.

• "Consider the order of your food. Eat vegetables first, protein and fats second, and starches and sugars last. This allows starch and sugar to be absorbed less into the bloodstream, creating a smaller glucose spike."

The goal is to keep your blood sugar at relatively steady levels. Your glucose should normally not rise more than 30 mg/dl (1.7 mmol/L) after meals. If it does, you likely did not follow the three bulleted steps above or you overfilled your glucose fuel tank with too many carbs.

By following these suggestions, you should see a dramatic boost in your efforts to lose weight.

12. Don't Try to Lose Weight Too Quickly

When we need to lose weight, it's definitely a good idea to take the bull by the horns and go for it. The problem is, most people want to take not only the bull, but the entire herd by the horns, maybe even the entire farm, and get it done much too quickly. It's a bad idea because it doesn't work, and it will likely backfire.

There are other contributing factors involved, but if we eat 500 fewer calories per day than our bodies need, we will lose a pound a week. (3,500 calories equal one pound. Doing the math, [500 x 7 days a week = 3,500 calories a week, or one pound of weight.]) So, losing more than two pounds a week means a calorie deficit of more than 1,000 calories a day. Considering that most of us need, on average, about 2,000 calories a day, that's half of our caloric need. That may work for a day or two or a little longer, but eventually we will become malnourished from both a lack of calories and nutrients. That will likely lead to extreme fatigue and hunger, which will lead to rebound bingeing. Bingeing is not a good way to lose weight!!! And before your binge is over, you'll be shocked to learn that you regained the weight you lost and a couple more pounds to boot.

How much weight can you safely lose per week? The consensus is one to two pounds, maximum. The more slowly we lose weight, the longer it tends to stay off. But you may have heard of people losing eight or ten pounds in a week. You may think: Why can't I do that and just sustain that pace for several weeks or months? Understanding weight loss, you'll know that it's not possible.

When we first go on a diet, we tend to lose lots of weight over the first five to seven days, and especially if we've cut back on carbohydrates. That's because as our carbohydrate total drops, we'll quickly shed a lot of water weight. Carbohydrates make us retain water. (Notice the word "hydrate" hiding in the word "carbohydrate.") And water, as you know, is heavy. But that process happens quickly and once it's done, it's done. There's no more spare water to lose. From that point on, all that's left to lose is fat and the little bit of muscle that also tends to get burned in the process. That is a slow process; it takes time.

It likely took years to put on extra weight. But that doesn't mean that it needs to take years to get rid of it. If you work hard at it, and especially if you exercise patience and apply the points in this chapter, you should be able to safely, and sanely, lose one to two pounds a week, or 52 to 104 pounds a year. Be happy and content with small gains.

Do you need to lose weight? Go for it. Proceed slowly, steadily, patiently, and wisely. You can do this!

13. Avoid Yoyo Dieting

Yoyo. What a great name. It refers to the children's toy that goes up and down on a string on your finger and that was all the rage in the mid-twentieth century. Almost every child had a yoyo.

Yoyo dieting. What a bad idea. It refers to the crash dieting that causes weight to go down and back up and that almost every adult has been victim to at least a few times in their lives. The results have not been good. (Note: No one actually plans on yoyo dieting. Their plan is for their weight to go down and stay there . . . the problem is, before they know it, their weight rebounds and comes right back up again.)

What's the problem with yoyo dieting? Simply put, it does not work. It's also a health hazard. Typically, a yoyo dieter tries to lose weight too quickly, often by restricting their caloric intake to less than half of the calories (energy) that they need. They may sustain that for a few hours, days, or weeks, and then, when the body reaches the point of severe energy and nutrient lack, the diet is abandoned and so is self-control. The weight all comes back, very quickly, and frequently with extra "bonus" pounds included.

Even if someone was to escape a yoyo dieting episode without gaining additional pounds from their starting point, it's still a dangerous practice. Why? Longevity research leader Valter Longo reports that if someone loses more than ten percent of their body weight even twice in their lives, that person will have increased health problems and a reduced life expectancy.

Dr. Joel Fuhrman describes this process beautifully in his book, which is fittingly entitled *The End of Dieting*. He writes:

> A 1993 study examined the correlation between weight cycling and obesity in rats. Researchers restricted the caloric intake of one group of rats and kept a second group of rats on their regular diet. When they put the first group back on its

regular diet, the rats in that group ended up with more body fat than the rats that were fed the same number of calories as part of their regular diet. The consistency of caloric intake made for a leaner rat, while the fluctuation of calories led to a fatter rat. The same holds true for humans. When we cut back our calories dramatically in the hopes of losing weight and then increase them once we reach our 'goal weight,' our lipogenic enzymes, the enzymes that store fat, shoot up. Such weight cycling is particularly harmful. It leads to more abdominal fat and visceral fat, the two types of body fat that place people at the highest risk of diabetes, heart disease, and cancer. Visceral fat is the fat under your abdominal wall. It surrounds your internal organs, engulfing your liver, intestines, kidney, pancreas, and heart with fat. Subcutaneous fat, on the other hand, is directly under your skin. It's the fat you can pinch. Visceral fat, which is deeper inside your belly, is associated with a number of serious health concerns, including high blood pressure, insulin resistance, diabetes, and heart disease. When you diet, you lose subcutaneous fat. But when you go off the diet and gain weight, you put on more visceral fat. It takes years to get rid of visceral fat. And it's almost never accomplished by crash dieting. Losing visceral fat requires a permanent commitment to healthy eating and healthy living through regular exercise. (Fuhrman)

Ted Naiman, author of the book *The P:E Diet: Leverage your biology to achieve optimal health*, sums this matter up nicely by counseling: "Do not 'go on a diet.' Start eating now the way you are going to eat forever."

That's one of the main keys to losing weight. Nutrient rich whole foods, long-term, slow and steady, is the optimal way to lose weight and to keep it off.

14. Exercise Helps, But It's Not Essential for Weight Loss

I wasn't sure if I should include this point in the book, because this is a book about nutrition. Exercise is not nutrition. However, this chapter is titled "How to Lose Weight Safely . . . And Keep it Off," and exercise is definitely a factor in weight loss. On that basis alone, I think it should be included, though very briefly.

Yes, exercise does help in the process of losing weight. Aerobic-type exercise is helpful, such as walking, running, swimming, skating, or biking. Those exercises raise the heart rate and metabolism, and therefore they burn calories. Resistance exercises, such as weightlifting and exercise bands, are helpful too. They build muscles, and increased muscle mass causes more calories to be burned.

That said, please know that it is possible to lose weight without engaging in significant exercise. The following saying has become popular in recent years: "Get fit in the gym, lose weight in the kitchen." And it's true, it works that way. Engaging in exercise brings many benefits to mind and body, including additional weight loss, but weight loss is not dependent on exercise. By controlling what you eat, how you eat, how much you eat, and when you eat, you can find much success in losing weight.

Let's revisit one of the opening quotes from the start of this chapter: *"Until you get your nutrition right, nothing is going to change."* So now you know how to get your nutrition right and how to lose weight. Practice everything in this chapter . . . and watch the excess body fat begin to drop off, slowly, but steadily. It's a thing of beauty when it happens, and it will happen right on schedule if you do the right things.

Chapter 28

"The Pleasure Trap"—Please Beware

"Quitting smoking is easy. I've done it a thousand times."—Mark Twain

• Why you can't stop eating the foods (or doing other things) that you know are harmful to you.

The pleasure trap? What is that??? You may not have heard of this trap before, but unbeknown to you, you may be very familiar with the trap itself. In fact, you may have been caught in it before, and you may even be stuck in it right now. Most people living in industrialized countries are. The pleasure trap is easy to fall into and difficult to get out of. We are surrounded by conditions that make landing in the pleasure trap common. This is a very bad thing, because the pleasure trap is damaging, and it can be deadly. This chapter will give you an overview of what the pleasure trap is, how it can harm you, how to avoid it, and how to climb out of it if you happen to fall into it.

First, a little background on the "pleasure trap." The term was coined by psychiatrist Doug Lisle and his longtime friend Dr. Alan Goldhamer, who is the founder of the renowned TrueNorth Health Center in Santa Rosa, California, USA. They explain the phenomenon in detail in their 2003 book *The Pleasure Trap, Mastering the Hidden Force that Undermines Health & Happiness,* which I highly recommend. In this chapter, I'll be providing a quick overview of the pleasure trap. I'll be including two graphics from the book *The Pleasure Trap,* which both Dr. Lisle and Dr. Goldhamer, as well as their publishing company, have graciously permitted me to display in this book.

So, what exactly is the pleasure trap? It's the biological and psychological process that causes one to fall into addictive or destructive behavior.

Let's take cocaine use as an example. Suppose a person has never used cocaine. But on one occasion they are tempted and try cocaine. What happens? Cocaine has a powerful effect on the pleasure centers in the brain. It absolutely lights up those centers, as massive amounts of pleasure hormones, such as dopamine, are produced right in the brain itself. What happens next? Of course, that person is likely going to want to feel that way again, and soon. So, cocaine dose number two soon follows. Pretty much the same effect occurs, perhaps to a slightly lesser degree, but the pleasure is still intense. Soon to follow is episode number three, then four, and so on. Cocaine is highly addictive, and in no time the person is hooked. They have to have their next hit of "coke" to feel right; they feel miserable without it.

However, in the process, their reaction to the drug has changed. When they started, they used cocaine to feel elated. But now, they need their next hit of cocaine not to feel elated, but to feel "normal." Because without cocaine, they feel sick and miserable. At this point, they are sad victims of the pleasure trap. They've become addicted to an unhealthy substance. Even though each dose of cocaine is damaging to them and potentially lethal, it actually feels "healthful," because without it, they feel incomplete or lacking; they feel blasé, weak, and sick. At first, cocaine use took them from feeling normal to elated. Now it takes them from feeling lousy to feeling normal again. So, the pleasure trap is essentially synonymous with addiction. Again, the term "pleasure trap" describes the process in which a person physically and psychologically becomes entwined in addictive or unhealthy behavior.

It's wise to avoid becoming addicted to any type of harmful substance, whether that be cocaine, heroin, tobacco, and so on. But the pleasure trap is more than about just drugs. It's also about food. Whether it's addiction to drugs or to food, the same exact mechanisms take place in the body and the brain.

Many, if not most, find themselves in the pleasure trap over their food choices. And the results can be just as deadly, long term, as those who are addicted to drugs. Millions and millions have died prematurely from being caught in the pleasure trap, and millions more have seen their health compromised or destroyed.

Elvis Aaron Presley and the Pleasure Trap

One stark example of a man who fell into the pleasure trap with food, as well as with other substances, was Elvis Presley. (I'm almost afraid to use Elvis as an example, for fear young readers might be asking, What's an Elvis Presley?) When Elvis was a young man, until perhaps his early 30s, he was known for his dashing looks, fine physique, energetic dancing, and seemingly unlimited energy. By the time he died at the age of 42, he was a completely changed man. He was grossly obese, had a huge stomach, was distorted and bloated, and his movement was severely limited. In just a few years, he had transformed from a picture of vibrant health to a picture of poor health. It was difficult to even watch him "perform." He could barely move, he tended to forget lyrics of songs he had sung for years, and he poured sweat profusely. What happened?

Elvis got caught in the pleasure trap. He became trapped into a lifestyle that he could not escape from, and it killed him. Elvis' drug use was notorious, but so was his diet. He craved the richest and most unhealthy foods imaginable. His favorite snack was peanut butter and banana sandwiches, fried in butter, washed down with several Pepsis. He ate a pound of bacon with breakfast every day as well as beef with every meal. He was known to go on intense food binges of pizza, ice cream, bacon, and cheeseburgers. According to Susan Doll, in her book *Elvis For Dummies*: "Rumours also claimed that he once ate 30 cups of yogurt, 8 honeydew melons, and a hundred dollars worth of ice cream bars in one night." She also wrote that "he ate so many Spanish omelets that he created an egg shortage in Tennessee."

From his ideal weight of about 170 pounds, in just a few years, Elvis ballooned to a reported 250 to 350 pounds at the time of his death. His cause of death is unclear, but it's often listed as a heart attack or even chronic constipation from a four-month bowel obstruction. He died, by the way, while using the toilet, having fallen off the seat either before or after he died.

I'm sorry to paint such a gruesome picture, but that is reality, and it's a reality that we want to avoid falling into, even in a more minor way. So, let's take a look at the mechanics of the pleasure trap. Then we'll discuss how to avoid the trap and how to get out of it if you find yourself ensnared.

The Mechanics of the Pleasure Trap

Please notice the two graphics. One is entitled "Drug Addiction and Recovery." The other is "The Dietary Pleasure Trap." You'll notice that the lines in the two charts follow the same exact curve. That's because the effect in the brain and body is the same with addiction to food and addiction to drugs. Let's walk through this process step by step. For the sake of simplicity, we'll follow the Dietary Pleasure Trap chart. But again, the drug addiction chart mirrors these same patterns precisely.

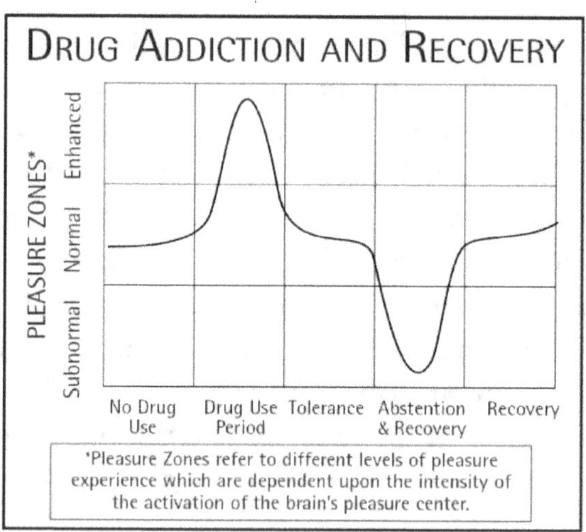

The Pleasure Trap, Goldhamer and Lisle, Book Publishing Company, 2003

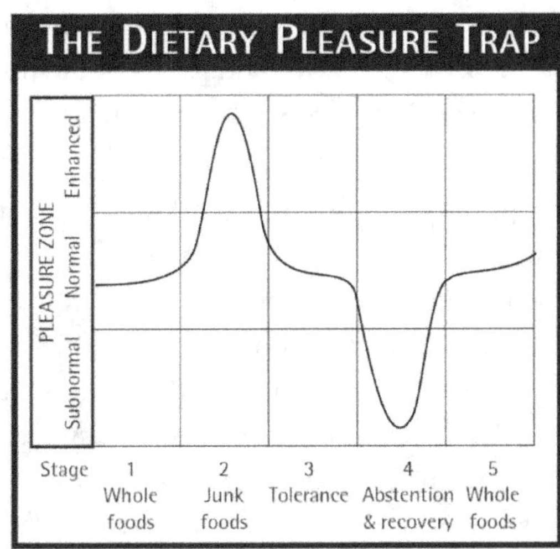

© The Pleasure Trap, Goldhamer and Lisle,
Book Publishing Company, 2003

Stage 1: Notice the person is eating a whole foods diet, and they are deriving a normal amount of pleasure from those foods. Those natural foods will taste good and be reasonably enjoyable and satisfying. This is, essentially, dietary life in its normal and healthy state.

Stage 2: The individual has begun to eat a steady diet of junk foods, such as fast foods, desserts, soft drinks, and the like. The pleasure in this stage will be exaggerated, or very high, as those foods will have an overwhelming effect on the pleasure centers in the brain—those foods will taste and feel "WOW!!!" Dopamine will be released in abundance.

Stage 3: This is the stage where the trouble becomes manifest—and this stage is reached quickly. The person is still eating those rich, unhealthy foods, but the brain has acclimated to the new diet, and the pleasure derived from the junk foods has dropped from enhanced back down to the normal zone. Dopamine is no longer released in high amounts from eating these foods. So now the person needs to eat those junk foods just to feel normal. They are enjoying food as much as they used to in stage 1, but the foods they are eating are damaging their health, whereas the whole foods they used to eat and derive as much enjoyment from were nourishing them. At this stage, they are caught in the pleasure trap. They are addicted, and regular wholesome foods just won't cut it anymore. (Have you ever heard someone say about a healthful salad: "I don't eat rabbit food!"?) Without rich junk foods, they'd feel sick. They've become dependent on them. And that takes us to the next stage . . .

Stage 4: The person realizes that they have to start to eat more healthfully. Perhaps their doctor told them to do so, or maybe their spouse or even their mirror or bathroom scale gave them a heads up. They return to a diet of healthy foods. What happens? Their pleasure zone drops way down to the bottom of the scale in the Subnormal category. In real life, this means they feel lousy—they are having withdrawal symptoms. The same healthy foods that used to make them feel normally satisfied after meals now leave them feeling devoid of energy and borderline sick, or in some cases really sick. (With drug addiction, the sickness of stage 4, withdrawal, can be extremely intense. Food addiction withdrawal is not as severe, but it is still quite unpleasant.)

Stage 5: Here's the good news . . . the human body and brain are very resilient and can recover. If that person continues to eat whole foods again for just a little while, maybe a couple of weeks or so, they will adjust and will again derive normal pleasure from those foods and will reap the benefits of a healthy diet.

The real trap is what happens at stage 2. You feel supercharged, as a new drug user will, and you want to continue to feel that way. The problem is: stage 3 is hiding right behind stage 2. You can't feel it coming, but come it will, quickly, and it will destroy your health. The longer you stay in stage 3, the more damage will be done to your health. And the sad thing is, you won't even feel good while it's happening. You'll need those rich junk foods just to feel decent. The wise move is to stay in stage 1, and if you ever get trapped and fall into stage 3, you'll need to pass through stage 4 and get to stage 5 and then remain there. Getting out of the pleasure trap takes work, but that work is temporary, and the benefits are long-lasting.

More on the Pleasure Trap

The pleasure trap works by creating artificial cravings. For instance, someone who is addicted to sugar will think that they are "hungry" when they are not. They don't need any more calories; what they need is the dopamine hit that comes from eating a sugary food, just like drug addiction. And your waistline does not care if you think you need that food or not. If it's excess calories, and especially in the form of sugar or other junk food, it's going to add to your fat stores no matter how much you feel like you "need" that food. (This is puzzling for many people. They believe that they are eating according to their appetite and not overeating. They may even be undereating, and yet they continue to gain weight. That prompts them to try a series of fad diets, and that only makes the problem worse.)

Along these lines, Dr. Joel Rosen, who is an adrenal specialist, notes something that I've seen over and over again. A person will say that they need a snack to raise their blood sugar. As Dr. Rosen puts it, 'their blood sugar probably hasn't been south of 100 mg/dl (5.6 mmol/L) in more than a decade.' Their sugar at that time may even be 150 mg/dl (8.3 mmol/L) or more. What they feel a need for, is not the boost in their actual glucose levels, but the dopamine hit that sugar, the drug, supplies. It's not their body that is hungry, it's their brain, and it's hungry not for food; it's craving a dopamine hit. That's the pleasure trap.

Notice how nutritarian founder Dr. Joel Fuhrman, who believes that 60 to 80 percent of the U.S. population suffers from food addiction, explains this in his book *The End of Dieting*:

> People who are overweight struggle with sweets, fried foods, chips, and fatty meats in exactly the same way smokers and drug addicts struggle with cigarettes and cocaine. If you're overweight, chances are you're a food addict. You eat because you physically feel the need for food, not because your body has any biological need for additional calories. Addiction is a physical and psychological dependence on a substance or behavior. Initially, the substance or behavior satisfies a person, but it quickly turns to compulsion when he or she needs more, just to avoid the

discomfort or pain that follows. Food addiction is complex and involves the stimulation of the digestive apparatus, which results in the release of bile, enzymes, and hormones and removes waste from the liver, kidney and bloodstream. It also intimately involves dopamine in the brain. A primary neurotransmitter, dopamine regulates, among other things, motivation and feelings of pleasure. Regardless of the addiction, the brain acts in the same way. Concentrated calories like sugar and oil, for instance, produce within food addicts a surge in dopamine levels similar to the levels in people who abuse illegal drugs. (Fuhrman)

How strong is this addiction? Astoundingly strong. Please note these fascinating words from an article in *Scientific American*, September 11, 2023:

> Given the option, most rats will choose sugar instead of cocaine. Their lust for the carbohydrate is so intense that they will go as far as to self-administer electric shocks in their desperation to consume sugar. Rats aren't alone in this drive. Humans, it seems, do something similar. People who've had bariatric surgery sometimes continue to overindulge in highly processed foods, those made from white flour, sugar, butter, and the like, even if it means later enduring vomiting and diarrhea. Daily snacking on processed foods, recent studies show, rewires the brain's reward circuits. Cravings for tasty meals light up the brain just like cravings for cocaine do. (*Scientific American*)

The Huffington Post reported on one study that provided a startling figure. It reads: "Have you heard about the rats who found sugar or saccharin more tantalizing than cocaine? That's right, in a fascinating study, most of the critters studied—a whopping 94 percent—wanted sugar or saccharin, not cocaine." Clearly, food addiction and the pleasure trap are real, and they are nothing to take for granted or tolerate.

The authors of *The Pleasure Trap*, Drs. Lisle and Goldhamer, offer this wisdom:

> A lack of exercise and sleep, and the resultant paucity of endorphin and serotonin production, results in people not

feeling good even when they may be managing many of life's challenges quite well. Not feeling good is an instinctive signal for action. But when we are not feeling well, we are unlikely to make the connection that a lack of sleep, exercise, and good dietary choices are the causes. We are unlikely to identify coffee, chocolate, high-fat foods, late-night TV, and a lack of exercise as factors. Quite the contrary, we are likely to suspect that a pleasure deficiency is the cause. This would have been the case in our natural environment, as feeling bad would often have been the direct result of some failure in important pleasure-seeking tasks. Not feeling good will typically intensify our search for powerful pleasurable experiences. And this is why the pleasure trap is so deceptive and powerful. (Lisle and Goldhamer)

So, when we don't feel good, we are wired to take steps to feel better. But we need to be very careful and make wise choices. For instance, if we are craving sweets because of a lack of sleep, the solution is pretty obvious . . . get more sleep. It's obvious, but sadly, it's usually ignored. Many will instead grab an extra cup of caffeine or will reach for a sugary food. It's best, though, to solve the problem at its source and not look for an artificial means to keep on going. That can quickly put someone in the middle of the pleasure trap. And when do you need to exercise self-control the most? When the cravings are the highest.

Is the New Chef Really Better Than the Old One?

A couple of years ago, I read a funny story about a man who had been on a fast in a health clinic. I can't remember the source of the story, but I believe it may have been Santa Rosa, California based, which means it was either at the TrueNorth Health Center or at McDougall Health and Medical Center. It could have, though, been somewhere else.

The story went like this: A rather gruff man who was having metabolic health problems was talked into going to a clinic where he would be fasted for a few days, semi against his will. When he first checked in, to prepare for the fast, he was put on a diet for a couple of days of the clinic's healthy foods served in the cafeteria. He hated the food, and he vigorously complained about how tasteless everything was. Then he successfully completed the fast. After the fast, and before he checked out of the clinic, he had another meal or two in the same cafeteria. Before he left, he made the comment that although he didn't like any of the process that he went through, he was glad that at least, in the meantime, they found a chef who could cook tasty foods, which were much better than the ones he ate when he first checked in.

However, there was no new chef and no new foods. Same chef, same foods. What had changed? The fast helped to pull the man out of the pleasure trap. His taste buds were now more true, and he found pleasure in eating those whole, natural foods. The fast served the purpose of stage 4 of the pleasure trap.

My first wholistic doctor, back in the 1980s, was a man named Rob Krakovitz. He was way ahead of his time. A brilliant nutritionist even by today's standards, Dr. Krakovitz would always encourage me to "keep your diet clean." And that's really the point and the way to elude the pleasure trap. Learn to find pleasure in whole foods. Marty Kendall, a brilliant engineer specializing in nutrition, wrote these sage words: "Once you give your body the nutrients it needs without excess energy, all the 'bad' things fall away and become irrelevant. When we emphasize the good things that we need from food (i.e., the essential nutrients), all the 'bad' things are crowded out." So yes, emphasize good foods and fill your diet with them. Find pleasure in them.

Everyone who is trying to recover from drug addiction is given the same advice . . . fill their lives with pleasurable and healthful activities, such as cultivating close friendships, hobbies, exercise, and so on. To erase bad habits, we need to crowd them out with good habits. It's the same with avoiding the dietary pleasure trap or making our escape from it. Learn to eat and to love natural foods—and eat them before you become overly hungry. It takes a little effort, but it's very doable. And when you do this, you will be able to avoid the pleasure trap and its devastating effects.

The Recommended Healthy Approach for The Pleasure Trap

Avoid being in the pleasure trap at all costs. If you are not there, keep up your good work. If you are there, take steps to escape. Life outside the pleasure trap is better than life inside it, and in the long run, the outcomes of those in or out of the trap are strikingly different. Remember, Elvis Presley stayed in the pleasure trap for many years, and the results were disastrous.

According to the accompanying charts in this chapter, if you are in stage 1, stay there. If you are in stage 3, move through stage 4 to get to stage 5, which is, in reality, a return to stage 1. Going through the withdrawal of stage 4 is not easy, but it's a relatively fast process, and the benefits of doing so are outstanding. Good health to you!

Chapter 29

Stabilize Your Blood Glucose

"Living with rollercoaster blood sugars sucks—appetite, mood or energy levels are in the toilet!" Marty Kendall, Big Fat Keto Lies

"Eating cereal in the morning has become a habit for many of us, but as you've learned in these pages, a sweet breakfast is a ticket to a glucose roller coaster. Eating a savory one will help curb hunger, banish cravings, boost energy, sharpen mental clarity, and more for the next 12 hours." Jessie Inchauspé, Glucose Revolution: The Life-Changing Power of Balancing Your Blood Sugar

• **Keeping your blood sugar levels stable throughout the day brings many benefits, including less hunger, fewer cravings, better mental clarity, less fatigue, more energy, better weight control, better mood stability, better hormone balance, less premature aging, less cognitive decline, and less chance of developing serious diseases like type 2 diabetes. You'll learn how to stabilize your blood sugar levels in this chapter.**

There you have it, right in the lead quotes to this chapter . . . Having rollercoaster blood sugar levels "sucks" and will put your energy levels "in the toilet." (Quite the expressive and colorful writing, Marty!) And a sweet breakfast can kickstart this whole process, which includes excessive hunger, cravings, low energy, poor mental clarity, and more.

Generally, I like to write my own material and sprinkle in quotes from the most respected sources in the field. However, I recently read an entry in a newsletter that is so spot on that I'm going to reprint it in its entirety, with permission granted by the writer and publisher. The source is the California Center for Functional Medicine, from their September 2022 newsletter. I'm very familiar with this center, CCFMD. In fact, my wife and I are their clients. They are completely cutting edge when it comes to health, lifestyle, and nutrition.

7-Day Blood Sugar Reset

© 2022, California Center for Functional Medicine (September 2022 Newsletter)

"Many people experience symptoms of blood sugar imbalance on a daily basis. In the short term, these can include fatigue, cognitive impairment, mood instability, headaches, cravings, increased appetite, and more. Over the long term, blood sugar imbalances can lead to weight gain, acne, hormonal imbalances, premature aging, and severe dysfunction like type 2 diabetes, infertility, fatty liver, and cognitive decline.

"Rebalancing blood sugar and improving insulin sensitivity is actually not that hard! Over the next seven days, we encourage you to implement these simple changes. Add just one each day, stacking the habits so that by the end of the week, you are a master of balancing your blood sugar.

"1. Have a high-protein breakfast. Aim to consume 20-30 grams of protein to improve blood sugar control throughout the rest of the day. Then, aim for at least 4-5 oz of protein per meal for the rest of the day.

"2. Take a 30-minute walk after meals. This helps move the glucose in your body after you eat to your muscles, lowering circulating blood glucose levels. If you do not have time for a walk after every meal, try to walk after at least one meal per day.

"3. Implement Time Restricted Eating (TRE). TRE is an eating pattern in which eating is limited to a certain number of hours each day. For example, with an eating window of 8 hours a day, the remaining 16 hours per day are spent fasting. TRE can help lower fasting and postprandial glucose levels, as well as decrease fasting insulin, and improve insulin sensitivity. Try starting with just 12 hours overnight. If you have your last meal finished by 7 pm, you won't eat again until 7 am. Gradually expand this time window.

"4. Always eat carbohydrates with protein, fat, and/or fiber. This helps slow the absorption of carbohydrates into the bloodstream, preventing a large spike in glucose after eating.

"5. Incorporate resistance training. Maintaining healthy skeletal muscle mass helps support insulin regulation and sensitivity. Skeletal muscles can take up circulating glucose to create cellular energy to fuel the body.

"6. Consume Vitamin K2 foods. Vitamin K2 helps to normalize blood glucose levels. This includes foods like natto, sauerkraut, liver and other organ meats, beef, pork, egg yolks, chicken, and fatty fish.

"7. Consider the order of your food. Eat vegetables first, protein and fats second, and starches and sugars last. This allows starch and sugar to be absorbed less into the bloodstream, creating a smaller glucose spike."

End of Newsletter

Concerning point number two, if you don't have the time for a 30-minute walk after each meal, a good alternative may be to take a 5 to 10-minute walk after most meals. Just that little bit of gentle use of the muscles will burn some of the glucose in the muscles and prevent the incoming meal from excessively raising blood glucose levels.

Of course, one of the most important aspects of keeping your blood sugar levels stabilized is to avoid eating too much of the foods that raise them. At the top of that list is carbohydrates, and in particular sweet and starchy carbs. By keeping your carbohydrate intake at moderate levels, or even low levels if necessary, and focusing on carbs that are slow glycemic, you'll be ensuring, along with the other tips mentioned in this chapter, that your blood sugar levels will remain relatively steady throughout each day. By doing this, you'll reap the following health benefits: less hunger, fewer cravings, better mental clarity, less fatigue, more energy, better weight control, better mood stability, better hormone balance, less premature aging, less cognitive decline, and less chance of developing serious diseases like type 2 diabetes—along with all of the other problems that presents.

Stability, when it comes to blood sugar levels, is a very good thing!

Chapter 30

Toxic Hunger. What is it, and Why is it Harmful?

• It's a sad fact that people often believe they are hungry when they are not. This causes them to eat to satisfy that "hunger." But eating when we are not truly hungry is self-defeating, and it will pack on unnecessary pounds and cause other health problems.

We may feel that we are hungry when we are not. At least, we are not hungry with true hunger, where our bodies need more calories and nutrients. This process can be very confusing, frustrating, and destructive. Let's address it and clear it up now.

The sensations of hunger can be caused by many things. Just the aroma from walking past the open door of a bakery might trigger hunger, or even the sight of the bakery might do it. Let's face it, a conversation about the bakery or even a memory of it may too!

You may remember or have heard about the scandal with subliminal advertising some years ago. It was found that some movie theaters, in particular drive-ins, had inserted very brief and nearly imperceptible frames of food items into movies at key points, perhaps showing a hot dog and soda. It happened so fast that the viewers couldn't recall seeing a thing out of the ordinary, but their subconscious mind picked up on it. When theaters did this, guess what happened at the food stand? Yep, hot dog and soda sales suddenly jumped minutes later.

I'll never forget something I read by Dr. Broda Barnes, who was an early leader in the field of endocrinology. He wrote a book called *Hope for Hypoglycemia*, and in that book, he described an experiment where subjects were injected with insulin, which would lower their blood sugar, and then the subjects were studied. Dr. Barnes did this experiment on himself, and he reported that soon after his injection he became so ravenously hungry that he 'would have eaten a fried doorknob.' Now that's hungry!

Today, most of us aren't injecting ourselves with insulin or being subjected to subliminal advertising, so what's going on? Dr. Joel Fuhrman, a brilliant nutritionist, explains it this way:

> The typical Western diet is characterized by high-calorie processed foods, oils, sweeteners, and animal products and is low in phytochemicals and other micronutrients. There is evidence that such a diet, low in micronutrients and phytochemicals, results in inflammation, oxidative stress, and accumulation of toxic metabolites.
>
> When digestion is complete, the body begins to mobilize and eliminate waste products, causing uncomfortable symptoms. If we allow waste metabolites to build up by eating unhealthy foods, we will feel discomfort when the body attempts to mobilize and remove these wastes. I propose that these sensations are actually symptoms of detoxification and withdrawal from an unhealthy diet, lacking in crucial micronutrients. I call this Toxic Hunger. Scientists now know that unhealthy food has effects on the brain similar to those of addictive drugs. Healthy food does not produce withdrawal symptoms — when the body is given vegetables, fruits, beans, nuts and seeds, there is nothing to detoxify. (Fuhrman)

There may be other causes of false hunger, such as disorders of the HPA axis, where adrenal function is compromised. And blood sugar disorders can be a factor too. But with toxic hunger, basically, people are going through symptoms of detoxification and withdrawal. They don't like the feeling, and they know that they can stop it by refueling their systems with more of the same types of food. It seems like a great fix . . . temporarily. But in the long run, it just makes the problem worse and worse until things get completely out of control.

It's always sad to see someone in public who is so obese that they can't walk. Perhaps they are in a cart in a grocery store, and their weight may top 400 pounds. How did that happen? Very likely, it's not that person's fault. They were probably fed a diet that was lacking in nutrients but filled with overstimulating foods from their childhood on, and they have suffered the effects of toxic hunger for years, never knowing that they needed to break the cycle by eating a diet that is balanced in energy and rich in nutrients.

One more cause of toxic hunger has to do with our hormones. Those who eat rich, stimulating foods lacking in nutrients throughout each day have become accustomed to the adrenal hits from adrenaline and cortisol that those foods will trigger. Just like with drug addiction, when the high of the last hit begins to subside, shakiness, fatigue and other "hunger" symptoms set in. Furthermore, the pleasure hormone dopamine is involved. Those rich foods cause us to secrete the pleasure hormone dopamine, and we feel an increasing need for more dopamine when the hit from the last one drops off.

If you've ever thought: "I just ate two hours ago, and I ate a lot, so I know I shouldn't be hungry, but I am," please know what you are feeling is not true hunger, but toxic hunger. Those feelings of hunger, such as headaches, shakiness, and fatigue feel like hunger, but it is not true hunger.

What is true hunger? Dr. Fuhrman explains it this way: "The function of true hunger is to prevent the breakdown of muscle tissue for energy; true hunger is a signal that directs the body to the precise amount of calories needed to maintain a healthy weight." If you are only eating when you feel hungry, yet are packing on the pounds, that's a very good indication that toxic hunger is controlling your appetite.

The Recommended Healthy Approach for Toxic Hunger

The way to put an end to toxic hunger is to stop the toxicity. And the way to do that is to begin to eat a diet that is rich in nutrients and is lacking substances that are harmful. I'm pleased to say that by following all of the advice in this book, you should be able to control and eliminate toxic hunger in no time. The first step, though, is to understand that what you are feeling is not true hunger but is toxic hunger, and now that you've read this chapter, you are equipped with that information and are well on your way. For further information, I suggest reading the chapter "The Pleasure Trap"—Please Beware." That chapter describes the addictive mechanism that drives one into the realm of toxic hunger. Further, part 3 of this book, "The World's Most Healthful Diet—A Helpful Cheat Sheet," describes exactly what to eat, how to eat, and when to eat to prevent toxic hunger. When you follow those principles, you will begin to heal and build a healthier, trimmer body.

Chapter 31

The SAD (Standard American Diet)

"One thing is for certain: if you want to be sick . . . eat as much as you want . . . of anything you want . . . whenever you want . . . This is called the 'standard American diet.'" Dr. Peter Attia, Longevity Expert

• There are some awful diets out there, but the Standard American Diet (SAD) is probably the worst of all. The SAD has also been referred to as the Deadly American Diet (DAD). It has prematurely claimed millions of lives, and millions more are on "death row." It's turned us into the unhealthy and sick and bloated nation that we are today.

We tend to be attached to the cultures we grew up with. It just feels right. It's who we are. That's not necessarily a bad thing in most instances. But when it comes to dietary habits, depending on where and how we were raised, it can be a huge problem. Most of us have grown up in a culture of horrendous food choices, and in recent decades, with more fast foods and a quicker pace of life, it's only getting worse. Dr. Joel Fuhrman, when describing the SAD, said that "people are on a race to commit suicide." What a sad way to live . . . and die.

Peter Attia, quoted at the outset of this chapter, wrote this: "Put down the Cheetos. Quality matters as much as quantity. The elements that constitute the SAD (Standard American Diet) are almost as devastating to most people as tobacco when consumed in large quantities, as intended: added sugar, highly refined carbohydrates with low fiber content, processed oils, and other very densely caloric foods." You are almost as bad off on the SAD as if you were a heavy smoker of tobacco.

Dr. Attia used Cheetos as an example, but the SAD goes way beyond that. It's filled with fast foods, junk foods, snack foods, sugary foods, chemicals, and lots of other substances that do not promote health—they compromise it or even destroy it. A typical meal for many is a burger, fries, and a soda to wash it down, with maybe a piece of pie or cake for dessert. Healthwise, that is a disaster.

Marketing has a lot to do with the SAD. Marketing experts know how to make what is bad seem normal or even good. I think back to four products from my childhood and the crafty way they were marketed. They are Wheaties, Tang, Pillsbury Food Sticks, and Wonder Bread.

Wheaties was called "The Breakfast of Champions." The boxes featured the best-known athletes. We could all be great athletes if we just ate this cereal. Tang was a powdered sugar drink that was supposedly the beverage of astronauts, Pillsbury Food Sticks were the sugary food bars that those same astronauts ate on their trips to space, and Wonder Bread helped "build strong bodies twelve ways." By eating those foods, the youth of our generation were all going to grow up to be champion athletes, astronauts, and body builders. How did that work out?

We can't just assume that the foods being offered to us are safe. Commercial interests and politics have a lot to do with what is made available. Sadly, the dollar comes before health in the commercial world.

Not convinced? Read on.

What is Really in Our Foods?

Our diets are loaded with unhealthy substances, including too much sugar, too much flour, unhealthy oils, poor quality meats and produce, and the like. That point is made clear throughout this book. But there are other substances in our food supply that you probably will be shocked to learn about. Notice, please, this quote from David Raubenheimer and Stephen J. Simpson, the authors of the book *Eat Like the Animals*:

> Take, for example, ice cream, which can be made at home using just cream, sugar, and fruit or other flavoring. Now consider the ingredients commonly used in the manufacture of mass-produced, commercial ice cream: benzyl acetate, a chemical that is also used in soaps, detergents, synthetic resins, and perfumes, and as a solvent in plastics and resins; aldehyde C-17, also used in dyes, plastics, and rubber; butyraldehyde, which is derived from the fuel gas butane and also used in the manufacture of pharmaceuticals, pesticides, and perfumes;

piperonal, once used in hospitals to control head lice; ethyl acetate, also used in glues and nail polish remover. And the list goes on. (Raubenheimer and Simpson)

Mark Hyman wrote the foreword to Vani Hari's best-selling book, *The Food Babe Way*. In that foreword, he adds his own insight to the matter:

> Most of us are completely oblivious to what we are eating and its impact on our health and our world. We know little about how our food is grown; how our seeds are engineered; how our farming methods harm the soil, air, and water, and contribute to climate change and dead zones in our oceans. We are mostly unaware of the chemicals that are added to our foods and how the hormones, antibiotics, plastics, and toxins we eat in our everyday foods harm our bodies. How could we know that we are eating Silly Putty in our French fries and yoga mat softeners in our bread; or cancer-causing preservatives such as BHA and BHT, which have been banned in every country but ours, or that dyes and coloring agents in our macaroni and cheese may cause hyperactivity and behavioral problems in our children; or that natural flavors are made from ground up animal parts; or that common foods contain secretions from beavers' anal glands? (Hyman)

That passage goes on, but mercifully, I'll stop there. I've quoted the famed Valley Girls in one other place in this book, but I must do so again: Grody to the max! Can you believe that people eat this stuff?

Where in the World Can We Find Healthy Foods?

It does seem complicated, but it's really simple. They grow out of the ground and are raised on responsible farms. That's it. Our food supply in its natural state, unblemished by commercial endeavors, is a wonderful and amazing source of health-building foods. We just need to learn what those foods are and then learn how to prepare them and eat them. The bottom line is this: if our diets are filled with whole natural foods and perhaps some high-quality animal products, the more we'll avoid the traps of the SAD, the healthier we'll be, and the longer we will live.

The Recommended Healthy Approach for The Standard American Diet

Abandon it. This chapter is not like the others in this book, where positive information is presented and recommendations are made. There is nothing positive about the Standard American Diet. The purpose of this chapter is to show you how deadly the SAD is and to encourage you to step away from it quickly. By following the suggestions in this book, you'll be aligning with the principles of sound nutrition. Is making the effort worth it? Absolutely. And I wish you much success in your endeavors to eat a clean, natural, healthy diet that makes you look and feel your best.

Chapter 32

Do Calories Count? Are All Calories Equal?

● **Does the theory of "calories in, calories out," ring true? In other words, is our weight gain or weight loss a simple matter of matching calories eaten to our energy output? Or is there more to it? If you eat the right foods, can you eat them in unlimited amounts and not gain weight? Are all calories created equal, or do some have a greater effect on weight control than others?**

Not too many years ago, the prevailing theory regarding weight gain was simple. It was all about calories eaten versus calories burned. This theory is called "calories in, calories out." According to the theory, if you eat more calories than you burn, you will gain weight, and if you eat less calories than you burn, you will lose weight. Today, many experts are teaching something entirely different. They believe that it's all about the types of food you eat . . . specifically, if you keep your carbs down and your glucose levels low and therefore your insulin levels low, they believe you can eat lots of calories and not gain weight. Insulin, they say, is the "fat storing hormone," and as long as your insulin levels are low, you will not store fat and gain weight no matter how much you eat, within reason.

Further, there is some controversy about calories themselves. In other words, do all calories have the same effect on weight gain, or are some calories better than others? Let's take a look.

The Bomb Calorimeter

The what? Yes, there actually is a device called a bomb calorimeter. If you are really geeky, you can buy one on Amazon. But what is a bomb calorimeter? It's the device that is used to determine the number of calories in food. And how it works is pretty simple. A food item is placed in the device, and then that food is completely burned to nothing. The bomb calorimeter provides a readout of the total amount of energy that is released when each specific food is burned. That is the number of calories that food ~~provides~~ contains.

Notice that I crossed out the word "provides" and replaced it with "contains." That's because while that specific food item contains whatever calories are burned in the machine, that's not to say that food item actually provides those calories as energy to the body. There is much more to it. The bomb calorimeter is simple and is made of metal; our bodies are extremely complex and made of flesh and blood and organs and hormones and so on. Our bodies process calories much differently than the machine that assigns calorie totals to foods.

Let's Compare Two Foods

To get a better grasp on this, let's compare two foods with the same caloric count. For this example, we'll use 100 calories of soda and compare that with 100 calories of black beans.

The 100 calories of soda, which is about a cup, is essentially all sugar, about 25 grams. When you drink those 100 calories of sugar, they will be metabolized very quickly. Pretty much all of the 100 calories you consume will count as 100 calories in your body.

But notice the difference with the serving of beans. A side dish of beans, about 2.5 ounces, contains 100 calories. But let's take a closer look at how those 100 calories are processed by the human body.

The fiber content of that serving of black beans is 7.5 grams. That's 30 calories that the bomb calorimeter counts, but your body can't use as energy, because fiber is indigestible. The equation now looks like this: (100 calories − 30 calories of fiber = 70 net calories.) There are 11 grams of starch in the beans. But about three of those grams are resistant starch. You may recall that resistant starch is resistant to digestion, acting more like fiber than starch. Some, a little more than half, does not get digested. So you can subtract about eight more calories. So now our equation looks like this: (100 calories − 30 calories of fiber − 8 calories of resistant starch = 62 net calories).

That's great, but we aren't finished. There is also what is called the "thermic effect of foods" (TEF). This refers to the amount of energy (calories) used to digest and metabolize each of the three macronutrients. Guess which macronutrient has the highest thermic effect? Protein. And that serving of beans has eight grams of protein. The thermic effect of protein is about 25 percent. So now the finished equation is (100 calories – 30 of fiber – 8 calories of resistant starch – 8 calories from the thermic effect of foods = 54 net calories). That's right, the 100 calories from beans yields, as usable energy in the human body, only about half of the calories of 100 calories of soda.

You could take this comparison even further by noting that the fiber in the beans will help with slowing down the glycemic response, which is a further weight reduction aid. And the fiber and resistant starch are great for your microbiome. The beans are also packed with nutrients, especially folate and minerals, including hard to get minerals like magnesium, zinc, and potassium. And you even get a little shot of omega-3 fats. So, what you eat makes a huge difference . . . you can see the wisdom in reaching for a serving of beans, or some other healthful whole food, instead of a can of soda, which is just an empty and destructive sugar bomb, or any man-made or junk food.

The Recommended Healthy Approach Regarding Calories

Definitively yes, calories count. The amount of calories you eat is very important to your health and to your weight control. However, "calories in, calories out," as though calories are all that matters, is a gross oversimplification of the process. We want to make sure that the calories we eat are nutrient dense, packed with wholesome nutrients. If you strive to control how much you eat and what you eat, eating only as many calories as you need (or slightly less if you are trying to lose weight), and you make sure that your meals are relatively low glycemic and nutrient dense, you will likely be able to keep your weight in the range that you want it. Of note, this is exactly how Blue Zones residents and centenarians tend to eat. They eat low-glycemic nutrient-dense foods and moderate amounts of those foods. The benefits to them in vibrant health and longevity have been astounding.

Chapter 33

Carb Back-Loading

• Carb back-loading is a little-known strategy that some nutritionists believe helps us to eat more in harmony with our natural energy rhythms. It involves eating the majority of our carbohydrates later in the day, when our cortisol levels are naturally lower.

There is a relatively new strategy involving carbohydrates that's called Carb Back-Loading. It's also referred to as Carb Cycling, but there is another form of Carb Cycling that is different from this one, so to avoid confusion, in this chapter I'll refer to it as Carb Back-Loading. Interestingly, the two main sources of research I'm using for this section are nutritionist Lindsay Christensen and functional medicine specialist Dr. Alan Christianson. Almost identical pronunciation of the last name, different spelling.

Here's how carb-back-loading works: You eat a small amount of carbohydrates with your morning meal, you eat a more moderate amount of carbohydrates with your noon meal, and you eat a larger (but not too large) amount of carbohydrates with your evening meal. This way of eating supposedly works in better harmony with your cortisol levels, supplying less food energy when your cortisol levels are higher in the morning, and more food energy when your cortisol levels are lower in the evening. Dr. Christianson, who wrote the book *The Adrenal Reset Diet*, explains the success he has had using this approach:

> In my book, THE ADRENAL RESET DIET, I wrote about a clinical trial I conducted. Everyone who participated in the trial was at some stage of adrenal dysfunction. Those at every stage saw movement back to healthy cortisol rhythms, using the carb-cycling strategy. (Christianson)

And here is how Lindsay Christensen describes the benefits of this carbohydrate eating strategy:

> To experience more benefits from an increased carb intake, consider trying carb back-loading. Carb back-loading is an

eating practice in which you consume the majority of your carbohydrates with your evening meal, rather than spread throughout the day. This practice reduces blood sugar fluctuations over the day, which are harmful to HPA (Hypothalamic-Pituitary-Adrenal) axis function. It supports the synthesis of serotonin and melatonin in the evening, which may enhance sleep quality. (Christensen)

Both Lindsay Christensen and Dr. Christianson have mentioned that sleep quality will improve with carb back-loading. And sleep quality is very important to our overall health, including any attempts at weight loss. So you may want to give carb back-loading a try, regardless if you have a known adrenal situation or not.

Chapter 34

Antibiotics

● **Antibiotics are commonly prescribed to treat a variety of medical conditions. Once viewed as practically a cure-all, in recent years they have increasingly been described as dangerous. Should you avoid antibiotics, or should you take them, and if so, when?**

Antibiotics are drugs, and this book is really about nutrition, or food. However, we've already discussed prebiotics and probiotics, so it seems fitting to provide just a brief section about antibiotics, as they are definitely in the same realm or discussion.

Do antibiotics save lives? Yes! Do antibiotics wreck lives? Yes! These drugs fall into the category of "a time and a place for everything." So, when is the time to use antibiotics, and when is the time to shun antibiotics?

Let me start by saying that antibiotics are grossly over prescribed today. Sometimes they are prescribed for conditions they can't even help with. Antibiotics are properly used to combat bacterial based illnesses. But they have zero effect on viruses—and yet, they are, at times, mistakenly prescribed to fight viral infections.

In such cases, is there any harm in taking antibiotics when you don't need them? Yes. Let's put that in capital letters and throw in an exclamation point . . . YES! We've already sung the praises of prebiotics and probiotics. That's because they build up the microbiome in the gut, feeding and supplementing the wonderfully beneficial bacteria that live there, helping the digestive and immune systems to function better. Antibiotics, keeping in mind the first four letters of that word, work against the good gut bacteria, destroying some of it, damaging the microbiome. (The word antibiotic literally means "against life.") That is never a good thing. Antibiotics can wreak havoc on your microbiome.

What problems do antibiotics cause? Note this entry from the CDC (Center for Disease Control and Prevention) website:

When antibiotics aren't needed, they won't help you, and the side effects could still hurt you. Common side effects of antibiotics can include rash, dizziness, nausea, diarrhea, or yeast infections. More serious side effects include Clostridioides diffcile infection (also called C. diffcile or C. diff), which causes diarrhea that can lead to severe colon damage and death. People can also have severe and life-threatening allergic reactions. (CDC)

Furthermore, Dr. Joel Fuhrman believes that taking rounds of antibiotics as children is a major cause of colon cancer in adults decades after childhood use. And knowing what antibiotics do to the digestive system, this makes perfect sense. (My observation is that Joel Fuhrman is a nutritional genius, and everything he says makes perfect sense. By all means, check out his books.)

The CDC recommends antibiotic use for strep throat, whooping cough, and urinary tract infections. It classifies as a "maybe," antibiotic use for sinus infections, middle ear infections, and bronchitis and chest colds in otherwise healthy children and adults. It does not recommend antibiotic use for the common cold, runny nose, sore throat (except for strep), and the flu.

The Recommended Healthy Approach for Antibiotics

Antibiotics do have their place in medicine. But they should never be viewed casually. Antibiotics are powerful medicines. They have serious side effects, and antibiotics should only be taken when they are absolutely necessary, such as in the case of a bacterial infection causing serious illness. If you can refrain from taking antibiotics and can heal without them, that's preferable. But if a bacterial infection is so severe that it can be life-threatening or may cause substantial damage, it may be prudent to take a round for that. Use good judgment and consult with your health professional. And, IF you do need a round of antibiotics, please remember to take the entire round. There's a tendency to stop taking them when we feel better, but if the full round is not taken, and the infection is allowed to remain simmering at an undetectable level, it may come back quickly in a stronger and more resistant form and cause more problems than the original illness did.

Chapter 35

Eating for Heart Disease

• All of the nutritional principles in this book are designed to be heart healthy. However, what if you have already been diagnosed with heart disease. What are the nutritional options?

All of the nutritional principles outlined in this book are definitely considered heart healthy. One of the diets that I favor most and incorporate in my recommendations is the PAMM Diet (Pan Asian Modified Mediterranean Diet), created by cardiologist Stephen Sinatra. Dr. Sinatra allows for generous amounts of fats in the diet, up to about 35 percent of total calories, but focuses on the most heart-healthy fats, such as monounsaturated fats (olive oil and avocados), and omega-3s (fish oil, walnuts, flax seeds, chia seeds), while limiting saturated fats.

Dr. Steven Gundry, who has a huge media presence, is another well-known cardiologist who recommends a diet that includes generous amounts of healthy fats. In particular, he is a big proponent of eating copious amounts of olive oil.

There are other cardiologists, however, who believe that, to reverse existing heart disease, a very low-fat diet is necessary, with about ten percent of calories, or even less, coming from fat.* The two best-known proponents of these diets are probably Dean Ornish and Caldwell Esselstyn. Dr. Ornish has written multiple books about this subject, and Dr. Esselstyn's best known book is *Prevent And Reverse Heart Disease: The Revolutionary, Scientifically Proven, Nutrition-Based Cure.* Additionally, Dr. Ornish created a low-fat treatment program that is approved by Medicare.

If you have existing heart disease, you know how important it is to be treated with the best possible protocol. Which is that, the low-fat regimen or the one that allows for more dietary fat? Each individual will have to make that decision. For individuals without heart disease, I definitely favor the PAMM diet or similar diets, the ones that allow generous amounts of healthy fats. But if you have heart disease, I recommend that you dig deep to discern which diet will give you the best chance of staving off further complications or will even allow you to reverse existing heart disease.

* Very low-fat diets are usually higher in carbohydrates. That might not be advantageous for someone with diabetes or prediabetes.

Chapter 36

"Vitamin S" . . . Sleep's Effect on Your Diet

"A growing body of research suggests that the foods you eat can affect how well you sleep, and your sleep patterns can affect your dietary choices."
Anahad O'Connor, New York Times

• The quality of our sleep has a huge impact on both our diet and our overall health, affecting our mental, emotional, and physical well-being. Learn how to sleep soundly at night and further boost your health and nutrition.

The subject of sleep is not normally covered in a book about nutrition. But because sleep is so important to our dietary habits, I'm going to include it here, though briefly.

Did you notice the catch-22 in the opening quote? Mr. O'Connor stated an obvious truth and acknowledged a vicious cycle. When we don't eat the right foods, we don't sleep well, and when we don't sleep well, we don't eat the right foods, and when we don't eat the right foods, we don't sleep well, and when we don't sleep well . . . That cycle may continue for years and even indefinitely.

Longevity expert Peter Attia makes the following observation: "A good versus bad night of sleep makes a world of difference in terms of glucose control. All things equal, it appears that sleeping just five to six hours (versus eight hours) accounts for about a 10 to 20 mg/dL (that's a lot!) jump in peak glucose response, and about 5 to 10 mg/dL in overall levels."

Ari Whitten, in his book *Eat for Energy*, makes the following profound statement: "Mitophagy (the removal of damaged cells) takes place during sleep. And if you don't get enough sleep, your body cannot get rid of the damaged mitochondria, and then you're functioning today on yesterday's poorly functioning and damaged mitochondria. And if that trend continues over months and years, chronically low energy is the unsurprising and logical result."

And Steven Gundry, a cardiologist who I've mentioned a few times in this book, makes the following observation in his book *The Energy Paradox: What to Do When Your Get-Up-and-Go Has Got Up and Gone*: "The importance of good-quality and sufficient sleep cannot be underestimated; it is as critical to our well-being as nutrition, yet it is often—to use a wheel analogy—the one spoke that is broken."

As these health professionals all point out, sleep is vital to our health, and it's tied inescapably to our nutrition.

What are Some Ways to Get a Better Night's Sleep?

Thankfully, there are some practical steps that can help people get a better night's sleep. Consider the following:

Melatonin. Melatonin is our sleep hormone: melatonin makes us sleepy and helps us fall asleep and stay asleep. Our levels of melatonin begin to rise in the evening and peak in the middle of the night. Then, just before we normally wake up, our levels begin to drop, and they stay very low during the entire day. Taking supplemental melatonin can help boost our levels of melatonin at the right time and make us sleepier, thus making it easier for us to fall asleep and stay asleep.

If you use melatonin, how much should you take? Normal doses are between 1 mg. and 10 mg. Each person reacts differently. For some, 3 mg. is excessive and creates discomfort, such as drowsiness the next day. For others, 3 mg. is not enough to have the desired effect. Our bodies make less than 1 mg. of melatonin per day. Therefore, start with 1 mg. or even less, see how that works, and consider adjusting from there. Please go low and slow with melatonin. It's a natural hormone, but that doesn't mean it's necessarily safe in doses that are too high for your body. Time-released melatonin will stay in your system longer and help you to stay asleep.

White noise machine. One of the biggest sleep disruptors is noise, and especially intermittent noise. If intermittent noise, such as traffic sounds, sirens, neighbors, family members, pets, etc. tend to disturb your sleep, you may find that a little machine that produces a steady noise, such as a fan sound or a waterfall sound, will drown out that noise and permit you to continue to sleep undisturbed. Those who prefer complete silence might find earplugs to be more helpful.

Deep breathing. Deep breathing activates the vagus nerve, which is part of the parasympathetic nervous system. Vagus nerve activation is calming and relaxing, which can promote sleep. Try to spend a few minutes breathing deeply and slowly before bedtime, focusing your attention on the process. You may find that your feeling of sleepiness increases in just a few moments of time.

Stretch. Gentle stretching is very relaxing, calming, and it also activates the vagus nerve. Don't bounce when you stretch, which can actually tighten muscles, but get into a comfortable stretch and hold it for about 30 seconds to a minute. While you are stretching, pay attention to the muscles that are being stretched in each particular pose. If during the stretch you begin to feel any pain, it's good to back off a little. Conversely, you may decide in the middle of a stretch that it would be advantageous to increase the stretch just a little. Be flexible, relax, and enjoy the process.

Control Blue Light. Blue light is a high energy light that is emitted from screens, such as smartphones, tablets, computer monitors, and televisions. Blue light pollution is a recent phenomenon, and it's a definite sleep enemy. It interferes with melatonin production, leaving people without the hormone they need most when they need to go to sleep. It's best to avoid all sources of blue light for at least one to two hours before you plan to go to sleep. You can also wear blue-light blocking glasses at night, which will protect your output of melatonin. There are also helpful apps for smartphones and tablets that reduce the amount of blue light emitted from the screen.

Blackout curtains. Light promotes wakefulness and darkness promotes sleep. Today's world is littered with too much light at night, and that has had a very detrimental effect on sleep. Consider getting blackout curtains, which prevent any light from coming in through windows. These curtains may not be the most beautiful things in the world, but they are very effective at promoting a good night's sleep, which in itself is a thing of beauty. As an alternative to blackout curtains, consider wearing an eye mask.

Don't eat too close to bedtime. We don't usually realize it because it takes place "behind the scenes," but digesting food is a huge task for the body. And our brains are involved in everything we do, including digesting food. Both our bodies and brains need complete rest while we sleep. Just as we don't want to be exercising or working while we are sleeping, we also don't want to be digesting significant amounts of food. It's best to stop eating at least three hours before you go to bed. If you must have something to eat closer to bedtime, try to keep it to a very light snack.

Keep regular hours. We have been gifted with wonderful circadian rhythms. These rhythms keep us going and keep us on schedule. Perhaps our most striking circadian rhythm is our sleep/wake cycle. We're programmed to be awake and active during the day and asleep at night. Our hormones literally synch with our circadian rhythms, and if we hold to a steady schedule, our hormonal patterns become very precise. By keeping regular hours, going to sleep and waking at about the same time each night and day, you'll be living in harmony with your hormones and circadian rhythms, which will help you to sleep better and to be more alert and more at peace.

Relaxing nighttime routine. Most of us can't just walk in the bedroom, jump in bed, and fall asleep. It takes some time for our bodies and our minds to adjust. And we can reduce that time period if we have a regular relaxing routine before we go to bed. Some like a warm bath, others may like to read relaxing material, others may gently stretch, still others may prefer listening to peaceful music. Find whatever works best to relax you. Doing so alerts your brain and body that you are preparing to sleep, which will reward you by slowing down the release of cortisol and enhancing the release of sleep-inducing melatonin. Your brain waves will begin to slow, your muscles relax, your nervous system will become calm, and . . . sweet dreams!

Don't exercise late at night. Exercise is generally sleep promoting. However, because exercise is stimulating, it works against sound sleep if done too close to bedtime. It's best to refrain from exercising for at least a couple of hours before you go to sleep. Rather, this is the time to get ready for your relaxing nighttime routine. Some find a slow, gentle walk may be sleep inducing before bedtime, but remember, this is not the time for powerwalking. Gentle stretching is also sleep inducing.

Natural herbs and substances. There are several herbs and other natural substances that have been proven to assist with sleep. Some of these are chamomile, GABA (not the same as the drug gabapentin), L-tryptophan, magnesium, valerian root, lavender, passionflower, L-theanine, hops. There is also an abundance of formulas containing some of these and other ingredients.

Over the counter meds. There are several OTC meds available that are known to help with sleep. These are generally gentler than prescription medications.

Prescription medications if necessary. If necessary, there are several prescription sleep medications that you can try. Please use these only as a last resort. Natural sleep is preferrable to medicated sleep. If you think you would benefit from using sleep medication, please consult with your health professional.

The Recommended Healthy Approach Regarding Sleep

Getting sufficient sleep is vital, but sleep can be easy to overlook and push aside for other activities. As Dr. Gundry mentioned, sleep may be the one spoke of our health wheel that is broken. And wheels without all spokes intact are dangerous. Resist this trend. Make quality and quantity of sleep a high priority. Your body and your brain will be glad you did. And it's an excellent way to improve your nutritional profile.

Part 3: The World's Most Healthful Diet—A Helpful Cheat Sheet

"Examining a range of nutrition research from studies in laboratory animals to epidemiological research in human populations provides a clearer picture of the best diet for a longer, healthier life." — *Top Longevity Expert and USC Leonard Davis School of Gerontology professor Valter Longo.*

• **This is your cheat sheet, if you will, to the world's healthiest diet. Follow these steps and you'll be amazed at the benefits you receive in the form of better, more vibrant health, including, if you need it, weight loss.**

Is there a healthiest diet in the world? I believe that there is, with variations allowed, and a few of the top nutritionists have pretty well nailed it in their recommendations. Among these are Mark Hyman, Valter Longo, Stephen Sinatra, Joel Fuhrman, and Dan Buettner. These authorities, who are all best-selling authors of health and nutrition books and true experts in the field, recommend almost identical diets with just slight variations. And they all line up with the diets of people who have the best records of health and longevity, including those who live in the

Blue Zones regions. Let's get to the highlights of this diet and way of eating.

I can sum up this section with the brilliant and oft-quoted words of Michael Pollan, who wrote: "Eat food. Not too much. Mostly plants." If everyone did that, there would be a huge jump in the overall health of the general public. Keep in mind that the first two words, "eat food," implies real food and not hyper-processed junk and fast food. Let's dig deeper and get into the specifics.

Note: This section is more or less a "cheat sheet" for your convenience. Everything that is included in this section is covered in greater detail in the previous chapters of this book.

1. **Your diet should feature vegetables.** Abundant vegetables are a key to a healthy diet. **Aim for at least five servings of vegetables a day.** Vegetables can be a combination of raw and cooked. Try to include a salad with green leafy vegetables every day. The majority of your vegetables should be non-starchy. Limit starchy vegetables to one or so servings per day, depending on your level of physical activity and your ability to control your glucose levels. If you are overweight, diabetic, or prediabetic, it would be helpful to have starchy vegetables less often, perhaps small amounts two or three times a week. (Starchy vegetables include potatoes, sweet potatoes, yams, butternut squash, cassava, corn, peas, etc.)

2. **You can include fruits in moderation.** Fruits are excellent foods, but they tend to be higher in sugar and have more glycemic impact than vegetables. **Aim for about one to two or perhaps three servings of fruit per day.** Focus on lower-glycemic fruits, such as berries. Especially be careful with the sugar in fruit if you have glycemic issues, such as diabetes or prediabetes, or you are trying to lose weight.

3. **You can eat beans and legumes.** These are healthful and staple foods of all of the Blue Zones, where people live extraordinarily long and healthy lives. Beans and legumes are also very economically friendly. **Aim for one-half to one cup of beans and legumes per day.** Make sure the beans are cooked properly, and if you make them at home, soak them

for at least eight hours before cooking. Consider including lentils, which many nutritionists favor over other bean varieties, in your diet.

4. **Eat healthy fats.** Don't be afraid to eat healthy fats. Contrary to a mistaken belief, fat in our diets does not translate into fat on our bodies or in our arteries; it's sugar and refined starches that make us fat and clog our arteries. **Aim for three to five servings of healthy fats per day, and have some fat with every meal.** Extra virgin olive oil, which is world-renowned for its healthful properties, including high levels of polyphenols, is an excellent choice. You can also include fatty fish, nuts, seeds, nut and seed butter, and avocados.

5. **You can eat nuts and seeds in moderation.** Nuts and seeds are little powerhouses of nutrition. Preferably, one or two of your daily fat servings should be from nuts and seeds. Walnuts, ground flax seeds, and chia seeds are notably high in heart-healthy omega-3 fats. Nuts and seeds are best eaten raw, but you can include some roasted nuts and seeds if you like. A serving of nuts and seeds is about one ounce, or one moderate handful. Because nuts and seeds are high in fat, it's important to eat them in moderation. Nuts and seeds, in moderation, are wonderful, healthful additions to the daily diet.

6. **You can include whole grains in your diet in moderation.** Grains are not the superfoods that they once were made out to be. They can spike sugar levels and there are issues with some modern grains, including rice and wheat. Still, whole grains can be a fine addition to your diet in moderation. **Aim to eat up to one or maybe two servings of whole grains in your diet per day.** An example of a serving of whole grains is ¼ to ½ cup steel cut oatmeal, ½ cup quinoa, or one slice of sprouted bread, such as Ezekiel Bread.

7. **You can include animal protein in moderation.** Research shows that animal protein does a better job at building and repairing muscles than plant protein. However, too much animal protein is not healthy. Make plants the dominant part of your diet, but use animal protein in small amounts to boost your amino acid profile. **You may aim to eat some form of animal protein preferably up to once daily. Some prefer a little more animal protein, especially if they have a need for muscular**

strength and power. Some may prefer animal protein less often, perhaps on just some days of the week. Older people, especially above age 65, require additional protein. Small servings of 20 to 30 grams of protein are sufficient, which equals about 4 ounces and is the size of a deck of cards or the average palm size. Fish is sometimes regarded as the healthiest animal protein. You can have other meats, such as poultry, and you can include red meat, perhaps once weekly.

8. **You can include dairy products, if you like, in moderation.** Dairy products have had an up-and-down reputation over the past several decades. Those who are lactose-intolerant or who otherwise react negatively to dairy products should not eat them. Others may eat dairy products in moderation. **If you eat dairy products, limit them to one or perhaps two servings a day.** Consider eating fermented dairy, such as yogurt and kefir, which provide beneficial bacteria to the intestinal tract and can help build a strong microbiome. Sheep and goat milk is superior to cow's milk, and if you drink cow's milk, milks with A2 protein are better than A1. (The milk commonly sold in supermarkets is A1.) Health food stores carry A2 milk. Better grocery stores may do so as well. The container will clearly indicate if the milk protein is A2.

9. **You can include eggs in your diet if you like.** Currently, many nutritionists favor eggs over dairy products. Eggs, while high in cholesterol, are low in saturated fat, are a good source of protein, and are loaded with nutrients. **Depending on your size and dietary needs, limit eggs to about seven a week.**

10. **Sweeteners should be used very sparingly.** It's best to learn to appreciate and enjoy the natural sweetness in foods. **If you do use natural sweeteners, such as honey or pure maple syrup, limit your use to one or two teaspoons a day. Stevia and monk fruit extracts are fine in small amounts. Sugar alcohols are best avoided. Artificial sweeteners are most often considered toxic. Avoid them.**

11. **It's important to drink sufficient pure water.** You are what you eat, and you are also what you drink. Our bodies are made up primarily of water, so it's important to cleanse and replenish with pure water. For this reason, drinking filtered water is recommended. Inexpensive water

filters do a reasonably good job but are limited; the more expensive filters remove fluoride. **Aim to drink at least half of your body weight (in pounds) in ounces of water a day. Example: If you weigh 200 pounds, drink at least 100 ounces of water a day.** You may find that drinking the majority of your water early in the day will prevent excessive nighttime urination. And it's best to not drink excessive amounts of water with meals, which can dilute the all-important digestive enzymes.

12. **Try to incorporate fermented foods.** Fermented foods are considered probiotics, and they are outstandingly beneficial to your microbiome, or gut health. Good gut health is extremely important to our overall health and well-being. **If possible, try to eat some fermented foods every day.** Examples of fermented foods are yogurt, kefir, sauerkraut (Bubbies brand is really good!), kimchi, kombucha, sourdough bread, miso, natto, fermented vegetables, torshi, apple cider vinegar, etc.

13. **Chew your food well.** Thorough chewing is one of the most important diet and health secrets I can share. Partially chewed food places stress on the digestive system and the entire body. Thoroughly chewed food leads to better digestion, better nutrient distribution, better glucose control, better weight control, and better overall health. **Aim to chew each mouthful of food between 30 and 60 times, reducing your food to a paste, to a liquid, or to the consistency of apple sauce.**

14. **Eat according to your circadian rhythms.** We have been blessed with an abundance of circadian rhythms. The most obvious of these involve the sleep/wake cycle. Our dietary habits can work with (or against) our natural circadian rhythms. Try to eat the majority of your calories earlier in the day, when you need more energy. Try to eat breakfast within an hour or two of rising. Don't eat too close to bedtime, which is when your body, including your digestive tract, needs complete rest. Usually, a period of three to four hours should elapse between your last meal or snack and when you go to bed, although some, such as those with blood sugar issues, may need to eat a light snack before bedtime. **And if you can, practice time-restricted eating,** which has been shown to provide remarkable health benefits. Time-restricted eating, which is

sometimes called "intermittent fasting," involves having a definitive eating period and a definitive non-eating period each day. Extreme fasting lengths are not necessary to achieve good health. Normally, a daily eating cycle of 10 to 12 hours and a fasting cycle of 12 to 14 hours is safe, sufficient, and effective at promoting health.

15. **Avoid unhealthy foods, such as most fast foods, junk foods, sugar, flour, deep fried foods, etc.** These "foods" can quickly wreck your health, and over the long term they can be devastating and even deadly. An English proverb says that we are "digging our own graves with a fork and spoon." Holistic health advocate Ann Wigmore wrote: "The food you eat can be either the safest and most powerful form of medicine or the slowest form of poison." Graves and poison are not good, and this book is in opposition to both of them! If you eat unhealthy foods, it's in your best interests to stop. If you need to slowly wean, gradually reduce the quantity of junk foods as you improve the quality of your diet. Crowd out the bad foods with the good foods that have already been discussed in this chapter.

Yes, you can still treat yourself to an occasional piece of pie, cake, ice cream, or whatever you desire—provided you can handle it and it will not lead you into a binge. But keep the serving small and get right back on with your healthy eating. We might eat for an hour a day, but we reap the benefits, or the consequences, of what we've eaten the other 23 hours . . . and then far into the future. Whatever it takes, make it your goal to eat as clean and healthy a diet as possible. It's worth it!

16. **Eat the highest quality foods you can afford.** If you can, buy organic produce. Seafood is best wild caught. Meats are best organic and free range, raised without antibiotics, which you don't want in your body. Beef is best "grass fed." Eggs are best when they are pastured, free range, organic, and possibly regenerative. Nuts, seeds, and grains are best organic, although I'd place a higher priority on obtaining organic produce. Try to buy produce in season if possible.

17. **Consider slight calorie restriction.** Overeating places an unnecessary strain on the body and leads to weight gain. It also

overwhelms and wears out your mitochondria—mitochondria is responsible for producing your body's energy. It's impossible to eat exactly the number of calories we need at each meal, so it's the course of wisdom to slightly, and I emphasize slightly, undereat. Those in the Blue Zones accomplish this by practicing the Japanese term hara hachi bu, which, when translated, means: "Eat until you're 80% full." If you need to lose weight, you should eat even fewer calories, but don't eat so little that you become weak, sick, overly hungry, or nutrient deficient. Aim to lose, at most, one to two pounds per week.

18. **Eat balanced meals.** Meals are healthier when they are balanced. A balanced meal is one that includes healthy amounts of protein, carbohydrates, fats, and fiber. It will also have a high nutrient density. A good protein will provide satiation and will provide the building blocks for body maintenance. The right amount of carbohydrates will provide the fuel you need. The right fats will help you absorb nutrients, provide satiation, and will bring other health benefits. And the fiber will help to fill you up and to slow the absorption of other carbohydrates, thus balancing your blood sugar. To be effective, those proteins, carbs, and fats need to be nutrient rich. An example of a balanced meal is four ounces of salmon, steamed vegetables with a tablespoon of olive oil, a slice of Ezekiel bread or half a sweet potato, and perhaps a small bowl of berries.

19. **Start your meals with vegetables, proteins, and fats. Then eat your carbs.** This practice helps you in two ways. First, vegetables will stretch your stomach and activate your stretch receptors, helping you to feel satiated sooner. Therefore, you'll be satisfied with less food. Second, the vegetables, proteins, and fats will slow the release of glucose from the carbs. This will lead to more stable glucose levels, which will lead to a host of benefits, including better weight control. NOTE: You don't have to save all of your carbs till the end of the meal. But it's a good idea to have some vegetables, proteins, and fats in your system before you begin eating carbs. "Naked carbs," as they are called, spike glucose levels quickly.

20. **Plant foods should dominate your diet.** Simply put, plant-based diets are the healthiest in the world. Plant-based does not mean that you can't eat meat, eggs, or dairy. It does mean that your diet is based, primarily, on plant foods. Plants are filled with nutrients, including fiber, that boost the body's systems in many ways. **For the best health outcome, aim to eat a diet that is at least 85-90 percent plants.** And of those plants, give preference to vegetables. The brilliant nutritional doctor Joel Fuhrman explains it this way: "Ninety percent of your daily diet should be made up of nutrient-rich plant foods, whose calories are accompanied by health-promoting phytochemicals: green and other non-starchy vegetables, especially mushrooms and tomatoes; fresh fruits; beans and legumes (including soybeans); raw nuts, seeds, and avocados; starchy vegetables; and intact whole grains."

21. **Supplement wisely.** Supplementation seems to be the course of wisdom in our stressful world. There are two reasons for this recommendation: 1. Modern farming methods, including soils that have been depleted of nutrients, are not supplying foods with the amounts of nutrients they used to have. 2. Stress depletes our stores of certain vitamins and minerals, increasing our need for replenishment. So, we need more nutrients than ever, but our food is supplying less than ever. Thankfully, we don't need to have a pantry filled with every supplement available. You don't need to overdo it, but your goal is to fill any lack that might be missing from your diet. **A good multi-vitamin/mineral, taken perhaps three or four times a week, and certain other key nutrients, such as magnesium, vitamin D, omega-3 fatty acids, vitamin C when under stress, and vitamin B12 if you are vegan, might be sufficient.** If you have any doubts about how to supplement for your individual needs, it's recommended that you consult a nutritionist or your medical professional (if that one has training in nutrition).

22. **Eat the rainbow.** This popular term refers to eating produce in all the different colors of the rainbow. **Or, simply put, eat produce with a variety of colors.** There's more to the color in food than just the aesthetics. Rather, each color brings with it certain specific nutrients that your body needs. For instance, orange produce is rich in beta carotene, potassium, lycopene, flavonoids, and vitamin C. By eating a wide variety

of colors, you'll be ensuring that you are getting most of the nutrients that you need. And yes, your salads will be much prettier!

23. **Customize your diet to your personal needs.** Writing that sentence scares me a little, because I don't want anyone to believe it means grabbing donuts because they think they need them. Rather, it means that while following all of the principles of a sound and healthy diet, each person will have unique needs and tastes. It's good to adjust to those, to a reasonable degree, of course. Each of the five Blue Zones is customized: each has its own local flare while still adhering to the principles that make a diet outstanding for health and longevity.

24. **Focus on nutrient density.** How fitting to end this section with nutrient density. Nutrient density is more or less an underlying theme of this book and of a healthy diet. Dr. Fuhrman created a very Einstein-like formula describing the importance of nutrient density: "$H = N/C$". That stands for "Health = Nutrients divided by Calories." In other words, the more nutrient dense our diet is, the healthier we will be. Simply put, nutrients build bodies. Eating foods with high nutrient values is a very smart thing to do.

Fun Note: I can't help but think of the coincidence involving point 24 and the great state of New Jersey. Albert Einstein was based in Princeton, New Jersey, and Joel Fuhrman's practice was in nearby Flemington, New Jersey. And that brings us to another New Jersey native, South River's Joe Theismann, star pro football quarterback and television analyst. Joe once made this comment, apparently while broadcasting a professional game: "Nobody in football should be called a genius. A genius is a guy like Norman Einstein."

Joe took a lot of flak for saying that . . . but he had the last laugh. Joe was referring to the valedictorian of his high school class, who was really named Norman Einstein. Norman, who his classmates considered to be brilliant, went to Rutgers University and studied physics, of course, and then he became a physician. Very, very clever, number 10.

My Favorite Nutritionists— Recommended Reading and Viewing

Throughout this book, I've quoted several of the best nutritional minds in the world. These men and women have done a wonderful job researching and sharing with us how we can live healthier, more satisfying lives. I'm happy to share their names with you, and I encourage you to look some of them up on Google, YouTube, Amazon, and the like. They provide a brilliant education.

I can't list the name of every excellent nutritional specialist here, but the following are some of those who I've paid particular attention to. I believe they have an outstanding grasp on the principles of sound and wise nutrition. Looking at the list, I can't help but notice that they are all on the same page nutritionally. Their teachings and conclusions are very similar. They get it!

Mark Hyman   Dr. Hyman is a nutritional genius. He's highly respected in the world of functional medicine by his peers, and for good reason. He is balanced and reasonable in his approach to nutrition, and he has written several excellent books. He's also widely available on YouTube. Dr. Hyman talks the talk and walks the walk—his biological age is reportedly twenty years younger than his literal age.

Joel Fuhrman   I love Dr. Fuhrman. He's produced an abundance of outstanding work in the field of nutrition, and he's the founder of the excellent and nutrient packed Nutritarian Diet. I highly recommend Dr. Fuhrman's books and videos to you. And to boot, Dr. Fuhrman is loaded with personality. He said something in an interview that was an impromptu attempt at humor, and he succeeded. My wife and I still giggle just thinking about it. Dr. Fuhrman was, in his youth, a champion figure skater, and at age 70, he is still very strong. As of a few years ago, I've seen videos of him jumping on tables from a standstill position. Maybe he's still doing so?

Valter Longo   USC-based Dr. Longo is often considered the top longevity expert in the world. He is closely associated with the Blue Zones, and I find his work to be spot-on, balanced, reasonable, and brilliant. His Longevity Diet is superb.

Dan Buettner   Dan Buettner is one of the few on this list who is not a medical doctor. He didn't need to be, because he was the perfect person to contribute to the field of nutrition as he has. As a member of *National Geographic*, Dan was assigned to study the Blue Zones regions, and he has done so in an outstanding way. He's shared the health secrets of long-lived Blue Zones residents with the world. Dan's teaching about nutrition is spot on and balanced.

Stephen Sinatra   Dr. Sinatra was a brilliant cardiologist and is the creator of the PAMM diet. I love his approach to heart health and nutrition. He is balanced, wise, likeable, and relatable.

Csilla Veress   Dr. Veress does not have a big media presence, but I know her work well and she is brilliant, warm, and compassionate. Her clients love her. And her grasp of the full scope of wholistic medicine is astounding and well-balanced. She works with the renowned TrueNorth Center in California, USA. Dr. Veress is a big proponent of time-restricted eating.

Marty Kendall   Marty Kendall is an Australian engineer who has devoted his life's work to the study of and teaching about nutritional health and longevity. In my opinion, he's done so beautifully and with great wisdom; he uses his engineering background to brilliantly conceptualize and explain nutritional principles. And his illustration of our four fuel tanks, which is shown in this book, is outstanding.

Linda Khoshaba   Dr. Khoshaba is a leader in the field of hormonal medicine. Her specialties are thyroid issues, such as Hashimoto's Disease, and adrenal health. Dr. Khoshaba is an endocrinologist, and she founded and directs Natural Endocrinology Specialists in Arizona, USA. My wife and I know Dr. Khoshaba, and we love her work. She is balanced, warm, compassionate, and very bright. She also made wonderful suggestions for the cover of this book! You can find videos on YouTube.

Will Bulsiewicz   Dr. B., based in Charleston, South Carolina, is a brilliant gastroenterologist. He is a foremost authority on the health of the gut microbiome. Dr. B. is ultra likeable and is an expert in diet and nutrition. His book, *Fiber Fueled: The Plant-Based Gut Health Program for Losing Weight, Restoring Your Health, and Optimizing Your Microbiome* is outstanding.

Izabella Wentz   Dr. Wentz is a thyroid and adrenal specialist. She's written top books about both thyroid health and adrenal health. Her approach to nutrition and wholistic medicine is balanced and reasonable.

Chris Kresser   Dr. Kresser has an amazing knowledge of all things health and nutrition. His web site is loaded with articles on almost every aspect of health and nutrition, and some have been known to use that site as their go-to resource for information. Dr. Kresser's wisdom shines through.

Steven Gundry   Dr. Gundry is a world-renowned cardiologist and has a huge presence on YouTube and in print. He's produced several excellent books. Dr. Gundry believes that lectins are very harmful, and he is a big proponent of the benefits of olive oil. I particularly like his book *The Energy Paradox: What to Do When Your Get-Up-and-Go Has Got Up and Gone*. Dr. Gundry, now nearing his mid-70s, by his own admission is cute . . . my wife and I agree.

Satchin Panda   Dr. Panda is a foremost authority on living in harmony with our circadian rhythms. His work is outstanding, and his knowledge and wisdom about the rhythms of life are remarkable.

Jessie Inchauspé   Jessie Inchauspé is the author of *Glucose Revolution: The Life-Changing Power of Balancing Your Blood Sugar*, which is an excellent guide that teaches how to lose weight by keeping your glucose levels balanced and steady.

This book is not opposed to a vegan diet, though I do believe including small amounts of animal proteins in the diet is beneficial for most people. If you are interested in the vegan lifestyle, there are excellent vegan (or near vegan) educators you can learn from. Here is a list of some of them:

Dean Ornish
Neal Barnard
John McDougall
Caldwell Esselstyn
Rip Esselstyn

Chef AJ
Alan Goldhamer
T. Colin Campbell
Pam Popper
Michael Klaper

Again, the names in this section are only a partial list. There are numerous experts who I know, and a more numerous amount of excellent nutritionists who I do not know, spread in localities throughout the country and the world.

Index

About the Author

David Klein is the author of several self-improvement books, focusing mainly on health and nutrition. He also developed a computerized program called Heart Risk Evaluations, which calculates the probability of heart disease based on multiple risk factors. The program was purchased by a medical group in Atlanta, Georgia, USA. David Klein has a deep interest and affection for logic—and he applies logic to his material, including health and nutritional science.

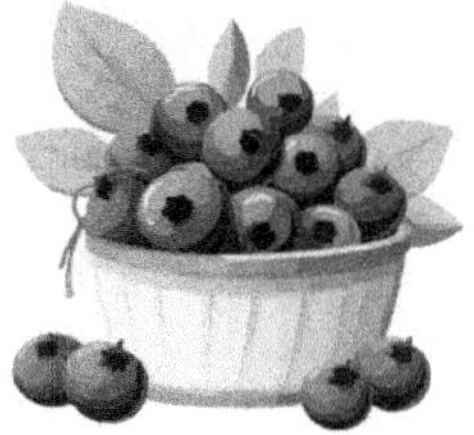